Basic
Ophthalmology

NINTH EDITION

Richard A. Harper, MD
Executive Editor

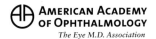
AMERICAN ACADEMY
OF OPHTHALMOLOGY
The Eye M.D. Association

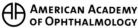
AMERICAN ACADEMY
OF OPHTHALMOLOGY
The Eye M.D. Association

American Academy of Ophthalmology
655 Beach Street
P.O. Box 7424
San Francisco, CA 94120-7424

Clinical Education Secretaries

Gregory L. Skuta, MD, *Senior Secretary for Clinical Education*

Louis B. Cantor, MD, *Secretary for Ophthalmic Knowledge*

Ophthalmology Liaisons Committee

Carla J. Siegfried, MD, *Chair*

Amy S. Chomsky, MD

Jo Ann A. Giaconi, MD

James W. Gigantelli, MD, FACS

Mary A. O'Hara, MD

Miriam T. Schteingart, MD

Samuel P. Solish, MD

Kyle Arnoldi, CO, COMT, *Consultant*

Mary Nehra Waldo, BSN, RN, CRNO, *Consultant*

Contributors, Ninth Edition

Richard A. Harper, MD, *Executive Editor*

Karla J. Johns, MD

David Sarraf, MD

J. Banks Shepherd III, MD

Carla J. Siegfried, MD

Academy Staff

Richard A. Zorab, *Vice President, Ophthalmic Knowledge, Clinical Education Division*

Hal Straus, *Director of Print Publications*

Barbara Solomon, *Director, CME, Programs, and Acquisitions*

Susan R. Keller, *Acquisitions Editor*

Kim Torgerson, *Publications Editor*

D. Jean Ray, *Production Manager*

Debra Marchi, CCOA, *Administrative Assistant*

Financial Disclosures

The authors and reviewers disclose the following financial relationships. **Carla J. Siegfried, MD:** (L) Allergan, (S) Pfizer. **Richard A. Harper, MD:** (C) Allergan.

The following contributors state that they have no significant financial interest or other relationship with the manufacturer of any commercial product discussed in their contributions to this book or with the manufacturer of any competing commercial product: Amy S. Chomsky, MD; Jo Ann A. Giaconi, MD; James W. Gigantelli, MD FACS; Karla J. Johns, MD; Susan Keller; Jacqueline S. Lustgarten, MD; Mary A. O'Hara, MD; David Sarraf, MD; J. Banks Shepherd III, MD; Miriam T. Schteingart, MD; Samuel P. Solish, MD; Kim Torgerson.

C = Consultant fee, paid advisory boards or fees for attending a meeting. L = Lecture fees (honoraria), travel fees, or reimbursements when speaking at the invitation of a commercial entity. S = Grant support.

First Edition, 1975; Second Edition, 1976; Third Edition, 1978; Fourth Edition, 1982; Fifth Edition, 1987; Sixth Edition, 1993; Seventh Edition, 1999; Eighth Edition, 2004.

Library of Congress Cataloging-in-Publication Data
Basic ophthalmology. — 9th ed. / Richard A. Harper, executive editor.
     p. ; cm.
  Includes bibliographical references and index.
  ISBN 978-1-61525-123-0
  1. Ophthalmology. 2. Primary care (Medicine) 3. Eye—Diseases—Diagnosis. I. Harper, Richard A., 1958- II. American Academy of Ophthalmology.
  [DNLM: 1. Eye Diseases—diagnosis. 2. Diagnostic Techniques, Ophthalmological. WW 141]
  RE46.B373 2010
  617.7—dc22
                                    2010027188
Printed in the United States of America
14 13 12 11 10   5 4 3 2 1

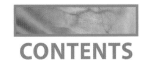

CONTENTS

FIGURES

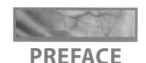

PREFACE

Basic Ophthalmology is designed to help the user obtain an appropriate ocular history and learn the examination techniques for a complete eye evaluation. From the history and clinical findings, the reader should be able to diagnose and manage or refer common ocular disorders. As in previous editions, the ninth edition features updated information and figures, as well as updated annotated resources. Where appropriate, tables are presented to summarize textual information and facilitate study.

The first edition of *Basic Ophthalmology* began in 1975 as a study guide in outline form. In contrast to earlier editions, the eighth and the current ninth editions place greater emphasis on historical information in evaluating visual complaints and assessing risk factors for ocular disease.

The U.S. population growth in the over-65 category is placing increasing demands on primary care providers to deal with age-related disease. Since many ocular disorders are more prevalent in this age group, primary care providers will need to have a solid understanding of the most commonly encountered disorders so that their patients will be effectively diagnosed, treated, and/or referred. To complicate this situation, there has been a decline over the past decade in the number of medical schools requiring a formal ophthalmology rotation, thus reducing the opportunity for medical students to obtain this essential information. Fortunately, many ophthalmology departments around the country are taking an active role in re-emphasizing the importance of ophthalmology in the medical student curriculum. *Basic Ophthalmology* provides an excellent resource for this effort, by establishing curricular content and later acting as a ready reference for practitioners encountering patients with ocular disorders.

This book can be used in a variety of settings. The concise presentation of information makes it ideal for brief ophthalmology rotations. If greater time is available, the resources can be consulted for more detail. This book is intended to be a flexible instrument that summarizes the important concepts, techniques, and facts of ophthalmology for nonophthalmic physicians and residents, especially those in primary care. The Ophthalmology Liaisons Committee anticipates that medical students will use this book in conjunction with comprehensive texts and other related resources annotated at the end of each chapter.

ACKNOWLEDGMENTS

Current contributors include Richard A. Harper, MD; Karla J. Johns, MD; David Sarraf, MD; J. Banks Shepherd III, MD; and Carla J. Siegfried, MD. The current contributors would like to thank their predecessors on the Medical Student Education Committee who partially through this book built a great foundation for medical student learning.

The following reviewed the eighth edition for currency, suggesting changes for the ninth edition: Karla J. Johns, MD; Jacqueline S. Lustgarten, MD; Mary A. O'Hara, MD; David Sarraf, MD; and Carla J. Siegfried, MD.

Special thanks to the reviewers of the revised manuscripts: Amy S. Chomsky, MD; Jo Ann A. Giaconi, MD; James W. Gigantelli, MD, FACS; Mary A. O'Hara, MD; Miriam T. Schteingart, MD; Carla J. Siegfried, MD; and Samuel P. Solish, MD.

WHO'S WHO IN EYE CARE

OPHTHALMOLOGIST

An ophthalmologist is a physician (doctor of medicine or doctor of osteopathy) who specializes in the medical and surgical care of the eyes and visual system and in the prevention of eye disease and injury. The ophthalmologist has completed 4 or more years of college premedical education, 4 or more years of medical school, 1 year of internship, and 3 or more years of specialized medical, surgical, and refractive training and experience in eye care. The ophthalmologist is a specialist who is qualified by lengthy medical education, training, and experience to diagnose, treat, and manage all eye and visual system problems and is licensed by a state regulatory board to practice medicine and surgery. The ophthalmologist is the medically trained specialist who can deliver total eye care (primary, secondary, and tertiary care services [ie, vision services, spectacles, contact lenses, eye examinations, medical eye care, and surgical eye care]), diagnose general diseases of the body, and treat ocular manifestations of systemic diseases.

OPTOMETRIST

An optometrist is a health service provider who determines visual acuity and prescribes spectacles and contact lenses. Optometrists may perform all services listed under the definition of optician. Optometrists are specifically educated and trained by an accredited optometry college in a 4-year course, but they do not attend medical school. There is state-to-state variation in education at optometry colleges. They receive a limited state license to examine the eye and to determine the presence of vision problems. Most states have passed legislation that permits optometrists to treat some eye conditions. This privilege varies from state to state. Some optometrists prescribe eye exercises for children with dyslexia and reading problems. (Thus far, the medical literature does not support the scientific efficacy of the treatment.) Payment for services of optometrists and ophthalmologists is equal. Medical boards generally do not have oversight of optometrists.

OPTICIAN

An optician is a professional who makes, verifies, delivers, and fits lenses, frames, and other specially fabricated optical devices and/or contact lenses upon prescription to the intended wearer. The optician's functions include prescription analysis and interpretation; determination of the lens forms best suited to the wearer's needs; the preparation and delivery of work orders for the grinding of lenses and the fabrication of eye wear; the verification of the finished ophthalmic products; and the adjustment, replacement, repair, and reproduction of previously prepared ophthalmic lenses, frames, and other specially fabricated ophthalmic devices.

TEST YOUR KNOWLEDGE

Test your present awareness about eye care by taking this quick true-false quiz. The test contains many statements that you may have heard before. Answers follow.

1. Reading for prolonged periods in dim light can be harmful to the eyes.   T   F

2. Children should be taught not to hold their books too close when reading, because doing so can harm their eyes.   T   F

3. Wearing glasses that are of the incorrect prescription can damage the eyes.   T   F

4. If children sit too close to the television set, they may damage their eyes.   T   F

5. Older people who may be having trouble seeing should not use their eyes too much because they can wear them out sooner.   T   F

6. People with weak eyes should rest their eyes often to strengthen them.   T   F

7. In time, children usually outgrow crossed eyes.   T   F

8. Contact lenses can correct nearsightedness, so that eventually neither contact lenses nor eyeglasses will be needed.   T   F

9. Children who have a problem learning to read are likely to have an eye coordination problem and can be helped with special exercises.   T   F

10. A cataract can sometimes grow back after cataract surgery.   T   F

11. A cataract has to be "ripe" before surgery can be done.   T   F

12. Nearsighted people become farsighted as they age, and farsighted people become nearsighted.   T   F

13. In older people, a sign of healthy eyes is the ability to read the newspaper without glasses.   T   F

14. People who wear glasses should have their vision checked every year to determine whether a change in prescription is needed.   T   F

15. Watching a bright television picture in a dimly lighted room can be harmful to the eyes if done for long periods.   T   F

16. Ideally, all people should use an eyewash regularly to cleanse their eyes.   T   F

17. A blue eye should not be selected for transplantation into a brown-eyed person.   T   F

18. In rare instances, a contact lens can be lost behind the eye and even work its way into the brain.   T   F

19. A cataract is actually a film over the eye that can be peeled off with surgery.   T   F

20. Headaches are usually due to eye strain.   T   F

TEST YOUR KNOWLEDGE: ANSWERS

1. False. Reading in dim light does not harm the eyes any more than taking a photograph in dim light would harm a camera.

2. False. Holding books close to the eyes to read is common in children, and no harm can come of it. Their eyes can accommodate (focus on near objects) easily and can keep near objects in sharp focus. In rare cases, holding a book close could be a sign of severe near-sightedness, which should be investigated; however, the habit of close reading itself will not cause nearsightedness in children.

3. False. Because glasses are placed in front of the eyes , they affect ight, not the eye. Looking through them cannot harm the eyes. However, an incorrect prescription may result in blurred vision, which can be uncomfortable.

4. False. Children with normal sight commonly want to sit close to the television set, just as they want to get close to reading material. This will not harm their eyes. Individuals will typically hold reading material or watch television at a distance that is comfortable for them.

5. False. The eyes are made for seeing. No evidence exists that using them for their purpose will wear them out.

6. False. Eyes that are "weak" for whatever reason did not become so from overuse, so they cannot be improved by rest.

7. False. Crossed eyes in children should always be considered serious; in fact, the condition requires referral to an ophthalmologist. Some children have apparent but not truly crossed eyes. In such cases, the apparent crossing is due to a broad bridge of the nose in young children. As the nose matures, this apparent crossing lessens and disappears. However, truly crossed eyes should never be ignored, as the condition will not improve with time.

8. False. Incorrectly fitted contact lenses can change the shape of the cornea but do not thereby correct myopia. Intentionally fitting contact lenses incorrectly to change corneal shape can cause permanent harm to the eyes.

9. False. The idea that reading problems are due to poor eye coordination is a misconception, as the results of many controlled studies have indicated.

10. False. Because a cataract is an opacity in the lens of the eye, the cataract cannot grow back when the entire lens is removed (intracapsular extraction). However, the posterior capsule of the lens may opacify when the lens capsule is left in place after removing the lens material (extracapsular extraction). This latter technique is nevertheless currently preferred because it best permits the placement of an intraocular lens implant; if posterior capsule opacity develops, it can be easily addressed with an outpatient laser procedure.

11. False. The need for cataract surgery is indicated principally by the degree of functional impairment caused by the cataract, not by any criteria related to its duration.

12. False. All individuals become presbyopic as they age. Presbyopia is the gradual loss of the ability to accommodate (focus on near objects, and it occurs irrespective of the person's underlying refractive error.

13. False. The ability of older persons to read without glasses may show only that they have myopia in at least one eye with reasonably good visual acuity. The nearsightedness could be caused by a cataract. Despite this ability, the person could also have a serious ocular disorder that was not yet symptomatic, such as glaucoma.

14. False. Glasses do not affect the health of the eyes. As long as an individual is satisfied with the vision provided by the present glasses, routine tests to measure their glasses prescription are generally unnecessary.

15. False. As indicated in some earlier answers, the eye cannot be harmed by the way in which light enters it. The eye merely deals with light, regardless of contrast. Watching television with or without illumination is a matter of comfort rather than harm. An individual who finds the marked contrast of a bright television picture in a dimly lighted room uncomfortable should turn on a light, but neither situation will harm the eyes.

16. False. Eyewash should be used as infrequently as possible. As long as it is functioning properly, the eyes' natural lubrication system is adequate for cleansing them.

17. False. Only the cornea can be transplanted, and the cornea is colorless in all eyes. (The iris gives eyes their color.)

18. False. The conjunctiva prevents a contact lens from passing behind the eye.

19. False. A cataract is a loss of the transparency of the normal lens of the eye, not a "growth" or "film" that covers the eye. If the lens becomes opaque enough to significantly impair a person's functional vision, the lens can be surgically removed and replaced with an intraocular lens implant. Nothing is "peeled" away.

20. False. Headaches are not usually caused by ocular factors. You will find more detailed and specific rationales for these answers in the various chapters of this text and in the resources suggested at the end of each chapter.

The Eye Examination

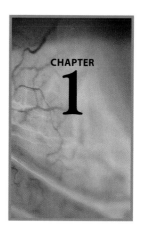

CHAPTER

1

OBJECTIVES

As a primary care physician, you should be able to recognize the significant external and internal ocular structures of the normal eye and to perform a basic eye examination. To achieve these objectives, you should learn to

- ➤ Elicit history and symptoms of ocular disease
- ➤ Recognize the essentials of ocular anatomy
- ➤ Identify anatomic changes of the eye due to aging
- ➤ Measure and record visual acuity
- ➤ Evaluate visual fields by confrontation
- ➤ Evaluate the eyelids
- ➤ Evaluate ocular motility
- ➤ Assess pupillary reactions
- ➤ Dilate the pupils when needed as an adjunct to ophthalmoscopy
- ➤ Use the direct ophthalmoscope for a systematic fundus examination and assessment of the red reflex
- ➤ Know when a referral to an ophthalmologist is necessary

RELEVANCE

The proper performance of a basic eye examination is a crucial skill for the primary care physician. Systematic examination of the eye enables the primary care physician to properly evaluate ocular complaints and provide either definitive treatment or appropriate referral to an ophthalmologist. Many eye diseases are "silent," or asymptomatic, while serious ocular damage is occurring. Obtaining a thorough history and performing a basic eye examination can reveal such conditions and ensure that patients receive the timely care they need. A basic eye examination may provide early warning signs of any of the following conditions: blinding eye disease, systemic disease, and tumor or other disorders of the brain. Important examples of irreversible blinding eye diseases that are potentially treatable if discovered early include glaucoma, diabetic retinopathy, macular degeneration, retinal detachment, and, in young children, amblyopia. Potentially vision-threatening or life-threatening systemic disorders that may involve the eye include diabetes, hypertension, temporal arteritis, and an embolism from the carotid artery or the heart. Tumor or other disorders of the brain may threaten both vision and life. Important examples include meningioma, aneurysms, and multiple sclerosis.

BASIC INFORMATION

An understanding of ocular anatomy, visual acuity, anatomic aging changes, and the patient's history all come into play when evaluating ocular complaints.

THE PATIENT'S HISTORY

When a patient presents to a primary care physician with ocular complaints, the first priority is to obtain a thorough ocular history. This is key in making the diagnosis and implementing a treatment plan.

Assessing Risk Factors for Ocular Disease

Obtaining a patient's systemic medical history and family ocular history is important for assessing a patient's risk factors for ocular disease. Just as with other body systems, reliable historical information allows the physician to more appropriately direct the physical examination. Areas to discuss include:

- Family history (blindness, glaucoma, ocular tumor, retinal detachment, strabismus, macular degeneration)
- Poor vision (excluding refractive error)
- History of eye trauma
- Medical history (diabetes mellitus, hypertension, hyperlipidemia, thyroid disease, autoimmune disease, malignancy)

Evaluating Visual Complaints

Knowing the onset, duration, and associated symptoms is invaluable in guiding the examiner to the correct diagnosis. Questions to ask include the following:

- Did the patient have prior good and equal vision in both eyes?
- Is the visual complaint monocular or binocular?
- Is central or peripheral vision affected?
- Is the change in vision acute or gradual?
- Is there any pain?
- Is vision distorted (metamorphopsia)?
- Is there double vision? In one eye or both (monocular or binocular)?

Greater detail is given in later chapters on historical information necessary to help diagnose specific ocular disease.

ANATOMY

Figures 1.1 through 1.4 show key external and internal ocular structures. Table 1.1 describes the principal structures of ocular anatomy.

ANATOMIC AGING CHANGES

A multitude of involutional aging changes can occur in the eye and adnexa. As the skin loses elasticity and succumbs to the effects of gravity, the brow sags over the superior orbital rim (brow ptosis). The levator aponeurosis, a tendinous

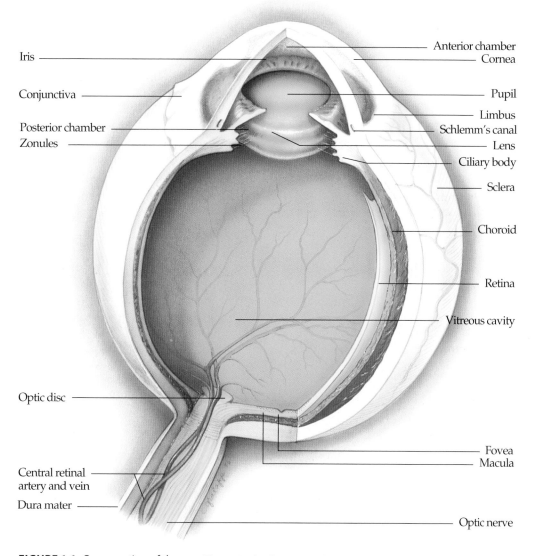

FIGURE 1.1 Cross-section of the eye. (Illustration by Christine Gralapp, MA, CMI)

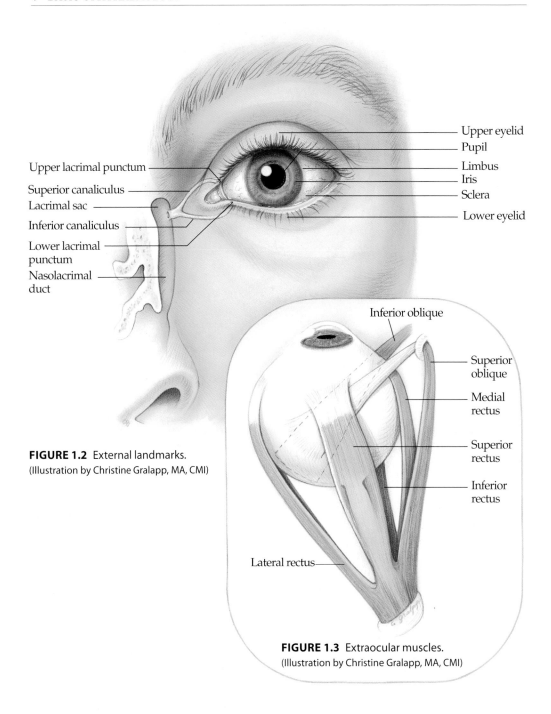

Upper eyelid
Pupil
Limbus
Iris
Sclera
Lower eyelid

Upper lacrimal punctum
Superior canaliculus
Lacrimal sac
Inferior canaliculus
Lower lacrimal punctum
Nasolacrimal duct

FIGURE 1.2 External landmarks.
(Illustration by Christine Gralapp, MA, CMI)

Inferior oblique

Superior oblique
Medial rectus
Superior rectus
Inferior rectus

Lateral rectus

FIGURE 1.3 Extraocular muscles.
(Illustration by Christine Gralapp, MA, CMI)

insertion from the levator muscle of the upper lid, may stretch or partially detach from the superior tarsal plate, allowing the upper eyelid to move closer to the visual axis and restrict peripheral vision (blepharoptosis, or, more commonly, ptosis). The lower lid suspensor ligaments likewise become lax, and the lid margin may rotate toward the cornea (entropion) or fall away from the globe (ectropion).

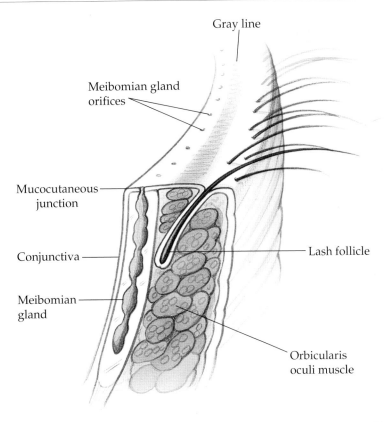

FIGURE 1.4 Eyelid margin anatomy. (Illustration by Christine Gralapp, MA, CMI. Reprinted from *Basic and Clinical Science Course*, Section 7: Orbit, Eyelids, and Lacrimal System. San Francisco, CA: American Academy of Ophthalmology, 2009–2010:143.)

Interruption of the normal lid architecture may predispose the patient to chronic tearing (epiphora) due to dysfunction of the lacrimal pump drainage mechanism (lid movement that normally propels tears toward the puncta). The lashes may be misdirected and rub on the cornea (trichiasis) independently or in conjunction with entropion.

The conjunctiva loses both accessory lacrimal glands and goblet cells over time, increasing the incidence of chronic dry eye. Older patients have likewise been shown to have a smaller tear lake. Of these patients age 65 and older, 15% to 20% report multiple persistent symptoms of dry eye, the severity of which can vary from mild irritation to debilitating pain and light sensitivity.

With advancing age, the crystalline lens continues to grow, crowding the anterior chamber angle and predisposing the patient to angle-closure glaucoma, particularly in the hyperopic patient with a narrow anterior chamber. The filtration of aqueous fluid through the trabecular meshwork slows, allowing a progressive increase in intraocular pressure and thus an increase in the incidence of open-angle glaucoma.

TABLE 1.1 Principal Structures of Ocular Anatomy

Eyelids	The outer structures that protect the eyeball and lubricate the ocular surface. Within each lid is a tarsal plate containing meibomian glands that empty at the eyelid margin. The lids join at the medial and lateral canthi. When the eyes are open, the space between the 2 open lids is called the *palpebral fissure*.
Cornea	The transparent front "window" of the eye that serves as the major refractive surface.
Sclera	The thick outer coat of the eye, normally white and opaque.
Limbus	The junction between the cornea and the sclera.
Conjunctiva	The thin, mostly transparent, vascular mucous membrane covering the inner aspect of the eyelids (palpebral conjunctiva) and sclera (bulbar conjunctiva).
Anterior chamber	The space that lies between the cornea anteriorly and the iris posteriorly. The chamber contains a watery fluid called *aqueous humor*.
Iris	The colored part of the eye that screens out light, primarily via the pigment epithelium, which lines its posterior surface.
Pupil	The circular opening in the center of the iris that adjusts the amount of light entering the eye. Its size is determined by the parasympathetic (constriction) and sympathetic (dilation) innervation of the iris.
Lens	The transparent, biconvex body suspended by the zonules behind the pupil and iris; part of the refracting mechanism of the eye.
Ciliary body	The structure that produces aqueous humor. Contraction of the ciliary muscle changes tension on the zonular fibers that suspend the lens and allows the eye to focus from distant to near objects (accommodation).
Posterior chamber	The small space filled with aqueous humor behind the iris and in front of the anterior lens capsule.
Vitreous cavity	The relatively large space (4.5 cc) behind the lens that extends to the retina. The cavity is filled with a transparent jelly-like material called *vitreous humor*.
Optic disc	The portion of the optic nerve visible within the eye. It is composed of axons whose cell bodies are located in the ganglion cell layer of the retina.
Retina	The neural tissue lining the vitreous cavity posteriorly. Essentially transparent except for the blood vessels on its inner surface, the retina sends the initial visual signals to the brain via the optic nerve. The retina, macula, choroid, and optic disc are sometimes referred to as the *retinal fundus* or, simply, *fundus*.
Macula	The area of the retina at the posterior pole of the eye responsible for fine, central vision. The oval depression in the center of the macula is called the *fovea*.
Choroid	The vascular, pigmented tissue layer between the sclera and the retina. The choroid provides the blood supply for the outer retinal layers.
Uvea	The vascular middle layer of the eye comprising the iris, ciliary body, and choroid.
Extraocular muscles	The 6 muscles that move the globe medially (medial rectus), laterally (lateral rectus), upward (superior rectus and inferior oblique), downward (inferior rectus and superior oblique), and torsionally (superior and inferior obliques). These muscles are supplied by 3 cranial nerves: cranial nerve IV, which innervates the superior oblique; cranial nerve VI, which innervates the lateral rectus; and cranial nerve III, which controls the remainder of the extraocular muscles.

The vitreous humor develops pockets of liquefied vitreous in the previously homogenous gel. This vitreous syneresis predisposes to a separation of the vitreous from its attachments to the retina and optic disc, called a *posterior vitreous detachment* (PVD). Since the vitreous is normally adherent to the retina, a PVD (Figure 1.5) in turn can predispose the patient to retinal traction, tears, and detachment.

Arteriosclerotic changes predispose the patient to vasculopathic cranial third, fourth, and sixth nerve palsies; retinal artery and vein occlusions; and anterior ischemic optic neuropathy.

The aging eye functions differently as well. Subjective testing in patients aged 50 or older sometimes reveals a loss of visual acuity, contrast sensitivity, and visual fields. Vertical smooth-pursuit eye movements and simultaneous vertical eye–head tracking decrease. Many older patients have trouble looking up, as well as moving the head up while simultaneously looking up with the eyes. Aging delays regeneration of rhodopsin, slows rod-mediated dark adaptation, and may lead to relative difficulty with night vision.

Aging does not condemn the elderly to a loss of functional vision, however. According to the Framingham Heart Study, an ongoing investigation of cardiovascular disease, acuity of 20/25 or better was maintained in at least 1 eye in 98% of patients ages 52 to 64, 92% ages 65 to 74, and 70% ages 75 to 85. The Framingham study found that subjective changes with age include dryness, grittiness, fatigue, burning, glare, floaters, and flashes; in addition, older patients had an increased risk of falls.

The study also noted other changes: a loss of corneal endothelial cells, yellowing and opacification of the lens, a smaller and less reactive pupil, and condensation of the vitreous gel. Retinal traction and tears were noted, as well as age-related changes in the retinal vasculature, and fewer neural cells in the retina and visual cortex.

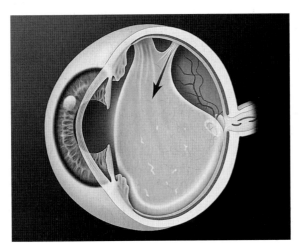

FIGURE 1.5 Posterior vitreous detachment. Partial collapse of the vitreous gel with a localized area of firm retinal adhesion and traction. (Illustration by Christine Gralapp, MA, CMI. Reprinted from Kassoff A. Flashes, floaters, and posterior vitreous detachment. *Focal Points,* Module 1. San Francisco: American Academy of Ophthalmology, 2003:4.)

OPTICS

The cornea and the lens are the refractive structures of the eye. The cornea provides approximately two-thirds of the refractive power of the eye, and the lens approximately one-third, to form an image on the retina. Reduced visual acuity will result if the axial length of the eye is either too short (ie, *hyperopia*; also called *hypermetropia*) or too long (ie, *myopia*) for the refracting power of the cornea and lens. Visual acuity also is reduced if the refracting power of the cornea and lens is different in one meridian than in another (ie, *astigmatism*). These optical defects can be corrected by the use of spectacles, contact lenses, or, in selected cases, refractive surgery. A pinhole placed directly in front of the eye will narrow the effective pupillary aperture and thereby minimize the blurring induced by a refractive error. Use of a pinhole device allows an examiner to estimate what a patient's visual potential would be with proper spectacle correction.

The ability of the ciliary muscle to contract and the lens to become more convex is called *accommodation*. With increasing age, the lens of every eye undergoes progressive hardening, with loss of ability to change its shape. Loss of accommodation is manifested by a decreased ability to focus on near objects (ie, *presbyopia*), while corrected distance visual acuity remains normal. Presbyopia develops progressively with age but becomes clinically manifest in the early to mid 40s, when the ability to accommodate at reading distance (35 to 40 cm) is lost. Presbyopia is corrected by spectacles, either as reading glasses or as the lower segment of bifocal glasses, the upper segment of which can contain a correction for distance visual acuity if needed. Some myopic patients with presbyopia simply remove their distance glasses to read, because they do not need to accommodate in an uncorrected state.

VISUAL ACUITY

Visual acuity is a measurement of the smallest object a person can identify at a given distance from the eye. The following are common abbreviations used in recording visual acuity:

- VA (visual acuity)
- OD (*oculus dexter*): right eye
- OS (*oculus sinister*): left eye
- OU (*oculus uterque*): both eyes

WHEN TO EXAMINE

All patients should have an eye examination as part of a general physical examination by the primary care physician. Visual acuity, pupillary reactions, extraocular movements, and direct ophthalmoscopy through undilated pupils constitute a minimal examination. Pupillary dilation for ophthalmoscopy is required in cases of unexplained visual loss or when fundus pathology is suspected (eg, diabetes mellitus).

Distance visual acuity measurement should be performed in all children as soon as possible after age 3 because it is a more sensitive test for amblyopia than those used in the recommended younger childhood eye evaluations (see Chapter 6). The tumbling E chart or another age-appropriate testing method is used in place of the standard Snellen eye chart.

ADDITIONAL TESTS

Depending on what the examination reveals and on the patient's history, additional tests may be indicated:

- Tonometry may be performed if acute narrow-angle glaucoma is suspected. The diagnosis of open-angle glaucoma requires more complex testing than simple tonometry.
- Anterior chamber depth assessment is indicated when narrow-angle glaucoma is suspected and prior to pupillary dilation.
- Confrontation visual field testing is used to confirm a suspected visual field defect suggested by the patient's history or symptoms; also used to document normal visual field.
- Color vision testing may be part of an eye examination when requested by the patient or another agency, in patients with retinal or optic nerve disorders, and in patients taking certain medications.
- Fluorescein staining of the cornea is necessary when a corneal epithelial defect (abrasion) or other abnormality is suspected.
- Upper lid eversion is necessary when the presence of a foreign body is suspected.

Details on how to perform both basic and adjunctive ocular tests appear in the next section.

HOW TO EXAMINE

Equipment for a basic eye examination consists of a few items that can be transported, if necessary, with other medical instruments (Figure 1.6). The slit-lamp biomicroscope is a stationary office instrument that augments the inspection of the anterior segment of the eye by providing an illuminated, magnified view. Standard equipment in an ophthalmologist's office, the slit lamp is also available in many emergency facilities.

DISTANCE VISUAL ACUITY TESTING

Distance visual acuity is usually recorded as a ratio or fraction comparing patient performance with an agreed-upon standard. In this notation, the numerator represents the distance between the patient and the eye chart (usually the Snellen eye chart, Figure 1.7). The denominator represents the distance at which a person with normal acuity can read the letters. Visual acuity of 20/80 thus indicates that the patient can recognize at 20 feet a symbol that a person with normal acuity can recognize at 80 feet.

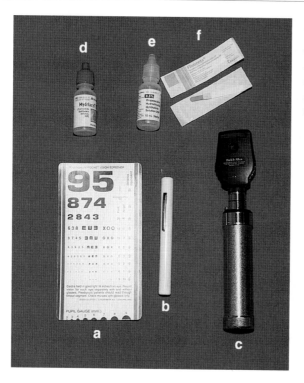

FIGURE 1.6 Equipment for a basic eye examination. **a.** Near vision card. **b.** Penlight. **c.** Direct ophthalmoscope. **d.** Mydriatic (dilating agent). **e.** Topical anesthetic. **f.** Fluorescein strips. (Courtesy Cynthia A. Bradford, MD)

Visual acuity of 20/20 represents statistically normal visual acuity. However, many "normal" individuals actually see better than 20/20—for example, 20/15 or even 20/10. If this is the case, you should record it as such. Alternative methods for recording visual acuity are decimal notation (eg, 20/20 = 1.0; 20/40 = 0.5; 20/200 = 0.1) and metric notation (eg, 20/20 = 6/6, 20/100 = 6/30).

Visual acuity is tested most often at a distance of 20 feet, or 6 meters. Greater distances are cumbersome and impractical; at shorter distances, variations in the test distance assume greater proportional significance. For practical purposes, a distance of 20 feet may be equated with optical infinity.

To test distance visual acuity with the conventional Snellen eye chart, follow these steps:

1. Place the patient at the designated distance, usually 20 feet (6 meters), from a well-illuminated Snellen chart (see Figure 1.7). If glasses are normally worn for distance vision, the patient should wear them.
2. By convention, the right eye is tested and recorded first. Completely occlude the left eye using an opaque occluder or the palm of your hand; alternatively, have the patient cover the eye.
3. Ask the patient to read the smallest line in which he or she can distinguish more than one-half of the letters. (If the tumbling E chart is being used, have the patient designate the direction in which the strokes of the E point.)
4. Record the acuity measurement as a notation (eg, 20/20) in which the numerator represents the distance at which the test is performed, and the denominator represents the numeric designation for the line read.

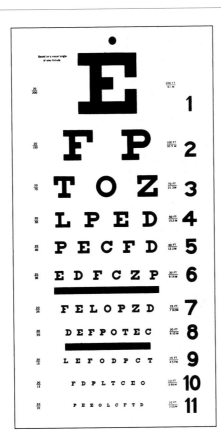

FIGURE 1.7 Snellen eye chart.

5. Repeat the procedure for the other eye.
6. If visual acuity is 20/40 or less in one or both eyes, repeat the test with the patient viewing the test chart through a pinhole occluder and record these results. The pinhole occluder may be used over the patient's glasses.

If a patient cannot see the largest Snellen letters, proceed as follows:

1. Reduce the distance between the patient and the chart. Record the new distance as the numerator of the acuity designation (eg, 5/70 if the patient is 5 feet from the chart and is only able to see the 20/70 size letters).
2. If the patient is unable to see the largest Snellen letter at 3 feet, hold up 1 hand, extend 2 or more fingers, and ask the patient to count the number of fingers. Record the distance at which counting fingers is done accurately (eg, CF 1 ft).
3. If the patient cannot count fingers, determine whether or not he or she can detect the movement of your hand. Record a positive response as hand motion (eg, HM 2 ft).
4. If the patient cannot detect hand motion, use a penlight to determine whether he or she can detect the direction or the perception of light. Record the patient's response as LP with projection (light perception with direction), LP (light perception), or NLP (no light perception).

TABLE 1.2 Visual Impairment Versus Visual Disability

VISUAL IMPAIRMENT	VISUAL DISABILITY	COMMENT
20/12 to 20/25	Normal vision	Healthy young adults average better than 20/20 acuity.
20/30 to 20/70	Near-normal vision	Usually causes no serious problems, but vision should be explored for potential improvement or possible early disease. Most states will issue a driver's license to individuals with this level of vision in at least 1 eye.
20/80 to 20/160	Moderate low vision	Strong reading glasses or vision magnifiers usually provide adequate reading ability; this level is usually insufficient for a driver's license.
20/200 to 20/400 or counting fingers (CF) 10 ft	Severe low vision; legal blindness by US definition	Gross orientation and mobility generally adequate, but difficulty with traffic signs, bus numbers, etc. Reading requires high-power magnifiers; reading speed reduced.
CF 8 ft to 4 ft	Profound low vision	Increasing problems with visual orientation and mobility. Long cane useful to explore environment. Highly motivated and persistent individuals can read with extreme magnification. Others rely on nonvisual communication: Braille, "audio books," radio, etc.
Less than CF 4 ft	Near-total blindness	Vision unreliable, except under ideal circumstances; must rely on nonvisual aids.
NLP	Total blindness	No light perception; must rely entirely on other senses.

Visual Impairment Versus Visual Disability

The term *visual acuity impairment* (or simply *visual impairment*) is used to describe a condition of the eyes. *Visual disability* describes a condition of the individual. The disabling effect of impairment depends in part on the individual's ability to adapt and to compensate. Two individuals with the same visual impairment measured on a Snellen eye chart may show very different levels of functional disability. Table 1.2 summarizes the differences between visual impairment and visual disability.

NEAR VISUAL ACUITY TESTING

Near visual acuity testing may be performed if the patient has a complaint about near vision. Otherwise, testing "at near" is usually performed only if distance testing is difficult or impossible—at the patient's bedside, for instance. In such situations, testing with a near card may be the only feasible way to determine visual acuity.

If the patient normally wears glasses for reading, he or she should wear them during testing. This holds true for the presbyopic patient in particular. The patient holds the test card—for example, a Rosenbaum Pocket Vision Screener (Figure 1.8)—at the distance specified on the card. This distance is usually 14 inches or 35 centi-

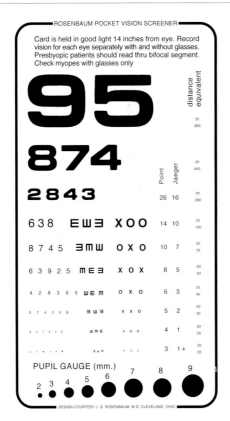

FIGURE 1.8 Rosenbaum Pocket Vision Screener.

meters. While the examiner occludes 1 of the patient's eyes, the patient reads the smallest characters legible on the card. The test is then repeated for the other eye.

Letter size designations and test distances vary. To avoid ambiguity, both should be recorded (eg, J5 at 14 in, 6 point at 40 cm). Some near cards carry distance-equivalent values. These are valid only if the test is done at the recommended distance. If a standard near vision card is not available, any printed matter such as a telephone book or a newspaper may be substituted. Both the approximate type size read and the distance at which the material was held are recorded.

VISUAL ACUITY ESTIMATION IN AN UNCOOPERATIVE PATIENT

Occasionally, you will encounter a patient who is unwilling or unable to cooperate with standard visual acuity testing or who may be suspected of feigning visual loss. Because the typical visual acuity test will not work for such a patient, you will need to be alert to other signs. Withdrawal or a change in facial expression in response to light or sudden movement indicates the presence of vision. A brisk pupillary response to light also suggests the presence of some degree of vision. The exception to this is the patient with cortical blindness, which is due to bilateral widespread destruction of the visual cortex. In almost all cases, referral to an ophthalmologist is recommended.

Chapter 6 discusses visual testing of infants and toddlers.

CONFRONTATION VISUAL FIELD TESTING

The examiner takes a position about 1 meter in front of the patient. The patient is asked to cover the left eye with the palm of the left hand; the examiner closes the right eye. Thus, the field of the examiner's left eye is used as a reference in assessing the field of the patient's right eye. The patient is asked to fixate on the examiner's left eye and then count the fingers of the examiner in each of the 4 quadrants of the visual field. Wiggling the fingers as a visual stimulus is not desirable. After the patient's right eye is tested, the procedure is repeated for the left eye, with the patient covering the right eye with the palm of the right hand, and the examiner closing the left eye.

AMSLER GRID TESTING

Amsler grid testing is a method of evaluating the functioning of the macula. (See Figure 3.18 and Chapter 3 for details.)

EXTERNAL INSPECTION

With adequate room light, the examiner can inspect the lids, surrounding tissues, and palpebral fissure. Palpation of the orbital rim and lids may be indicated, depending on the history (eg, trauma or mass lesion) and symptoms. Inspection of the conjunctiva and sclera is facilitated by using a penlight and having the patient look up while the examiner retracts the lower lid or look down while the examiner raises the upper lid. The penlight also aids in the inspection of both the cornea and the iris.

UPPER LID EVERSION

Upper lid eversion is sometimes required to search for conjunctival foreign bodies or other conjunctival signs. Topical anesthetic facilitates this procedure. The patient is asked to look down and the examiner grasps the eyelashes of the upper lid between the thumb and the index finger. A cotton-tipped applicator is used to press gently downward over the superior aspect of the tarsal plate as the lid margin is pulled upward by the lashes (Figure 1.9). Pressure is maintained on the everted

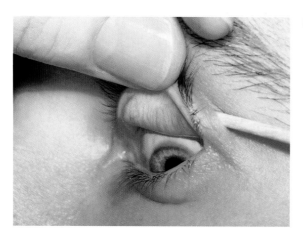

FIGURE 1.9 Upper lid eversion.

upper lid while the patient is encouraged to keep looking down. The examiner should have a penlight within reach to inspect the exposed conjunctival surface of the upper lid for a foreign body or other abnormality. A cotton-tipped applicator soaked in topical anesthetic can be used to remove a foreign body. To return the lid to its normal position, the examiner releases the lid margin and the patient is instructed to look up.

OCULAR MOTILITY TESTING

The patient is asked to follow an object in 6 directions, the cardinal fields of gaze. This enables the examiner to systematically test each muscle in its primary field of action (Table 1.3). Thus, a possible isolated weakness or paralysis of muscle can best be detected. (See Chapter 6 for a description of the cover test for the detection of strabismus, a misalignment of the 2 eyes, and for an illustration of the cardinal positions of gaze.)

PUPILLARY REACTION TESTING

Inspection of the pupils should be part of the physical examination. The patient's direct and consensual pupillary reactions to light are evaluated in a room with reduced illumination and with the patient looking at a distant object.

To test the direct pupillary reaction to light, first direct the penlight at the patient's right eye and see if the pupil constricts (a normal reaction). Repeat for the left pupil. To test the consensual pupillary reaction to light, direct the penlight at the right eye and watch the left pupil to see if it constricts along with the right pupil (a normal consensual response). Repeat for the left pupil, watching the right pupil for the response. Occasionally, this examination may reveal indications of neurologic disease. (See Chapter 7 for details on pupillary examination and a description of the swinging-flashlight test for the detection of an afferent pupillary defect in the anterior visual pathway.) Pupillary inspection may reveal active or prior ocular disease with alterations in pupillary shape or size that are the result of

TABLE 1.3 Cardinal Positions of Gaze

RIGHT AND UP	LEFT AND UP
Right superior rectus	Left superior rectus
Left inferior oblique	Right inferior oblique
RIGHT	LEFT
Right lateral rectus	Left lateral rectus
Left medial rectus	Right medial rectus
RIGHT AND DOWN	LEFT AND DOWN
Right inferior rectus	Left inferior rectus
Left superior oblique	Right superior oblique

local intraocular processes (eg, damage to the pupillary sphincter or adhesion of the iris to the lens).

ANTERIOR CHAMBER DEPTH ASSESSMENT

Usually, the anterior chamber is deep, and the iris has a flat contour. When the anterior chamber is shallow, the iris becomes convex as it is bowed forward over the lens. Under these conditions, the nasal iris is seen in shadow when a light is directed from the temporal side (Figure 1.10). As the shallowness of the anterior chamber increases, so do the convexity of the iris and the shaded area of the nasal iris. A shallow anterior chamber may indicate narrow-angle glaucoma (also called *angle-closure glaucoma*) or a narrow angle that could close with pupillary dilation, thus inducing an attack of angle-closure glaucoma. If a patient is suspected of having a narrow angle, he or she should not be dilated and should be referred to an ophthalmologist for evaluation.

To assess anterior chamber depth, follow these steps:

1. Shine a light from the temporal side of the head across the front of the eye parallel to the plane of the iris.
2. Look at the nasal aspect of the iris. If two-thirds or more of the nasal iris is in shadow, the chamber is probably shallow and the angle narrow.
3. If you are unsure of the extent of shadow, direct the light more from the front of the eye, which will eliminate shadows, and then return the light to the temporal side of the head.
4. Repeat the test for the other eye.

INTRAOCULAR PRESSURE MEASUREMENT

Intraocular pressure (IOP) is determined largely by the outflow of aqueous humor from the eye. The greater the resistance to outflow, the higher the intraocular

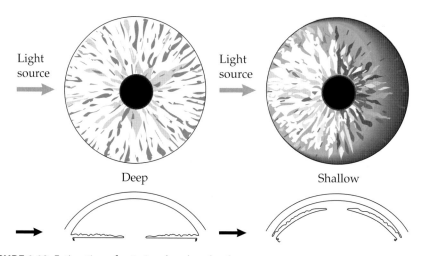

FIGURE 1.10 Estimation of anterior chamber depth.

pressure. Alterations in the actual production of aqueous humor also have an effect on the intraocular pressure.

Intraocular pressure varies among individuals. An IOP of 15 millimeters of mercury (mm Hg) represents the mean in a "normal" population. However, an IOP in the range from 10 to 21 mm Hg falls within 2 standard deviations of the mean.

Measurement of IOP is part of a glaucoma screening examination, along with ophthalmoscopic assessment of the optic cup. Diagnosing open-angle glaucoma requires additional testing not available to primary care physicians; therefore, IOP measurement is not indicated in this setting. However, IOP determination can be useful when the diagnosis of acute angle-closure glaucoma is being considered.

In the past, Schiøtz (indentation) tonometry has been an inexpensive and simple method for primary care physicians to measure intraocular pressure. A Schiøtz tonometer (if available and the physician is skilled in its use) can be used to measure the intraocular pressure in a patient with suspected angle-closure glaucoma. With the patient in a supine position, the Schiøtz device with a given weight is placed on the patient's anesthetized cornea and indents the cornea in an amount related to the IOP. A printed conversion table that accompanies the tonometer is used to determine the IOP in millimeters of mercury.

Currently, handheld electronic tonometers are available in some hospital emergency departments to measure intraocular pressure (Figure 1.11). These battery-operated devices can be used with the patient in any position, as opposed to other devices that require the patient to be either seated or supine. The intraocular pressure results are obtained rapidly with the electronic tonometer and correlate highly with those obtained by the Goldmann applanation tonometer (a slit-lamp–mounted instrument used by ophthalmologists) that is considered the gold standard for IOP measurement. Electronic tonometers are expensive and require daily calibration.

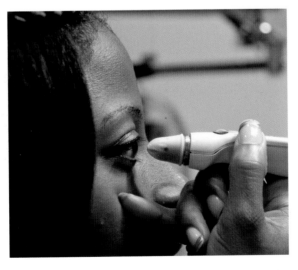

FIGURE 1.11 Electronic tonometry. Electronic tonometry can be performed with the patient in any position.

To perform electronic tonometry, the practitioner instills topical anesthetic in the patient's eyes, separates the lids, and gently applies the calibrated tonometer to the patient's cornea. The pressure reading and reliability rating displayed on the device are noted in the patient's record.

Topical anesthetics applied for tonometry have little effect on the margins of the eyelids. If the tonometer touches the lids, the patient will feel it and squeeze the lids together, impeding IOP measurement. This can be avoided by holding the patient's lids wide apart with the free hand while applying the tonometer tip with the other hand. Take care not to apply digital pressure to the eyeball while holding the lids apart, as it may produce a falsely high pressure reading. If the patient is wearing contact lenses, they must be removed before IOP is measured. Tonometry should never be attempted in a patient suspected of having a ruptured globe; doing so could result in further damage to the eye.

COLOR VISION TESTING

The normal retina contains 3 color-sensitive pigments: red-sensitive, green-sensitive, and blue-sensitive. A developmental deficiency in either the concentration or the function of 1 or more of these pigments causes various combinations and degrees of congenital color vision defects. Most such defects occur in males through an X-linked inheritance pattern. Color vision abnormalities also may be acquired in individuals with retinal or optic nerve disorders.

Color vision testing is performed with the use of pseudoisochromatic plates (eg, Ishihara plates), which present numbers or figures against a background of colored dots. The person with abnormal color discrimination will be confused by the pseudoisochromatic plates, which force a choice based on hue discrimination alone while concealing other clues such as brightness, saturation, and contours.

The patient should wear glasses during color vision testing if they are normally worn for near vision. The color plates are presented consecutively (to each eye separately) under good illumination, preferably natural light. Results are recorded according to the detailed instructions provided with the plates. Usually, a fraction is specified, with the numerator equivalent to the number of correct responses and the denominator the total plates presented. The type of color defect can be determined by recording the specific errors and using the instructions provided with the plates.

FLUORESCEIN STAINING OF CORNEA

Corneal staining with fluorescein (a yellow-green dye) is useful in diagnosing defects of the corneal epithelium. Fluorescein is applied in the form of a sterile filter-paper strip, which is moistened with a drop of sterile water, saline, or topical anesthetic and then touched to the palpebral conjunctiva. A few blinks spread the fluorescein over the cornea. Areas of bright-green staining denote absent or diseased epithelium (Figure 1.12). Viewing the eye under cobalt blue light (available on most direct ophthalmoscopes) or using a Wood lamp enhances the visibility of the fluorescence (Figure 1.13).

Two precautions to keep in mind when using fluorescein are

1. Use fluorescein-impregnated strips instead of stock solutions of fluorescein because such solutions are susceptible to contamination with *Pseudomonas* species.
2. Have the patient remove soft contact lenses prior to application to avoid discoloration of the lenses.

OPHTHALMOSCOPY

When examining the patient's right eye, hold the direct ophthalmoscope in the right hand and use your right eye to view the patient's eye. Use your left hand and left eye to examine the patient's left eye. The patient's eyeglasses are removed, and, barring large astigmatic refractive errors, most examiners prefer to remove their own glasses as well. Contact lenses worn by either patient or examiner may be left in place.

Pupillary Dilation

Pharmacologic dilation of the patient's pupils greatly facilitates ophthalmoscopy. Recommended agents include tropicamide 1% and phenylephrine hydrochloride

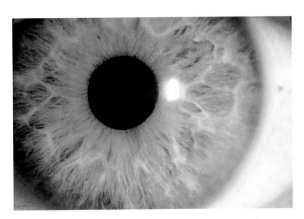

FIGURE 1.12 Fluorescein stain. A corneal abrasion is delineated by fluorescein stain, which marks any area denuded of epithelium. Irregularity of the corneal surface is indicated by the distorted light reflection.

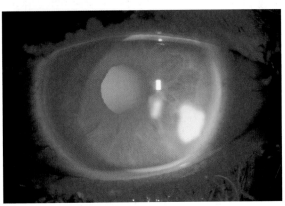

FIGURE 1.13 Fluorescein stain highlighted. The same eye in Figure 1.12 with the addition of cobalt blue light, which dramatically defines the corneal epithelial defect.

2.5% (see Chapter 9). Dilation of the pupil should not be done under the following conditions:

1. If assessment of anterior chamber depth suggests a shallow chamber and a narrow angle, do not dilate because an attack of angle-closure glaucoma might be precipitated.
2. If a patient is undergoing neurologic observation and pupillary signs are being monitored (eg, a head-injured patient), do not dilate until the neurologist or neurosurgeon determines it is safe to do so.
3. Dilation can cause blurred vision and light sensitivity for several hours, so patients must be informed of the potential impact on their activities such as reading and driving.

See Chapter 9 for instructions on applying topical agents.

Method of Direct Ophthalmoscopy

To perform direct ophthalmoscopy, follow these steps:

1. Have the patient comfortably seated. With the room lights dimmed, instruct the patient to look at a point on the wall straight ahead, trying not to move the eyes.
2. Set the focusing wheel at about +8. Set the aperture wheel to select the large, round, white light.
3. Begin to look at the right eye about 1 foot from the patient. Use your right eye with the ophthalmoscope in your right hand. When you look straight down the patient's line of sight at the pupil, you will see the red reflex (see the next section).
4. Place your free hand on the patient's forehead or shoulder to aid your proprioception and to keep yourself steady.
5. Slowly come close to the patient at an angle of about 15° temporal to the patient's line of sight. Try to keep the pupil in view. Turn the focusing wheel in the negative direction to bring the patient's retina into focus.
6. When a retinal vessel comes into view, follow it as it widens to the optic disc, which lies nasal to the center of the retina.
7. Examine the optic disc, retinal blood vessels, retinal background, and macula in that order (see the next section).
8. Repeat for the patient's left eye, holding the ophthalmoscope in your left hand and viewing with your left eye.

Red Reflex

Light reflected off the fundus of the patient produces a red reflex when viewed through the ophthalmoscope at a distance of 1 foot. A normal red reflex (Figure 1.14) is evenly colored, is not interrupted by shadows, and is evidence that the cornea, anterior chamber, lens, and vitreous are clear and not a significant source for decreased vision. Opacities in the media—such as a corneal scar, cataract, or vitreous hemorrhage—appear as black silhouettes and can be best appreciated when the pupil has been dilated. Most retinal pathology will not affect the red reflex.

Optic Disc

In most cases, when viewed through the ophthalmoscope, the normal optic disc (Figure 1.15) is slightly oval in the vertical meridian and has a pink color that is due to extremely small capillaries on the surface. Detail of these small vessels cannot be discerned, which differentiates them from pathologic vessels on the optic disc. The disc edge or margin should be identifiable (sharp). A central whitish depression in the surface of the disc is called the *physiologic cup*. The optic disc can be thought of as the yardstick of the ocular fundus. Lesions seen with the ophthalmoscope are measured in disc diameters (1 disc diameter equals approximately 1.5 mm).

A great deal of normal variation exists in the appearance of the optic disc. The size of the physiologic cup varies among individuals. (See Chapter 3 for a discussion

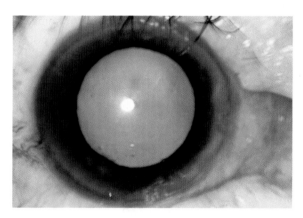

FIGURE 1.14 Red reflex. Reddish light reflected from the fundus can be visible even at a distance of 1 or 2 feet when the direction of illumination and the direction of observation approach each other—a condition that can be achieved with the ophthalmoscope.

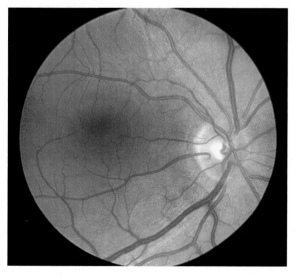

FIGURE 1.15 Normal fundus. A normal optic disc is shown, with a small central physiologic cup and healthy neural rim. Major branches of the central retinal artery emanate from the disc, whereas the major branches of the central retinal vein collect at the disc. Temporal to the disc is the macula, which appears darker; no blood vessels are present in the center.

of glaucomatous cupping.) The pigmented coats of the eye—the retinal pigment epithelium and the choroid—frequently fail to reach the margin of the optic disc, producing a hypopigmented crescent (Figure 1.16, left). Such crescents are especially common in myopic eyes on the temporal side of the optic disc. Conversely, an excess of pigment may be seen in some eyes, producing a heavily pigmented margin along the optic disc (see Figure 1.16, right). The retinal nerve fibers (ie, ganglion cell axons) ordinarily are nonmyelinated at the optic disc and in the retina, but occasionally myelination may extend on the surface of the optic disc and retina, producing a dense, white superficial opacification with feathery edges (Figure 1.17).

Retinal Circulation

The retinal circulation is composed of arteries and veins, visible with the ophthalmoscope (compare Figure 1.15 with Figure 1.18). The central retinal artery branches at or on the optic disc into divisions that supply the 4 quadrants of the inner retina; these divisions lie superficially in the nerve fiber layer. A similarly arranged system of retinal veins collects at the optic disc, where spontaneous pulsation (with collapse during systole) may be observed in 80% of normal eyes. The ratio of normal vein-to-artery diameter is 3:2. Arteries are usually lighter in color

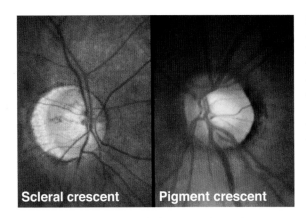

FIGURE 1.16 Scleral crescent and pigmented crescent. This figure shows normal variants of the optic disc. On the left, retinal and choroidal pigmentation does not reach the disc margin, leaving an exposed white scleral crescent. On the right, pigment accumulation is seen at the disc margin.

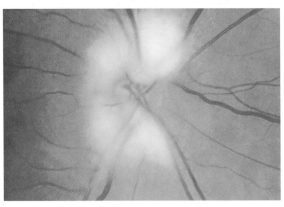

FIGURE 1.17 Myelinated nerve fibers. Usually, the axons of the retinal ganglion cells acquire myelin sheaths only behind the optic disc. Occasionally, as a variant, myelin is deposited along axons at the border of the disc or even away from the disc, elsewhere in the retina. These white, feathery patterns may be mistaken for papilledema.

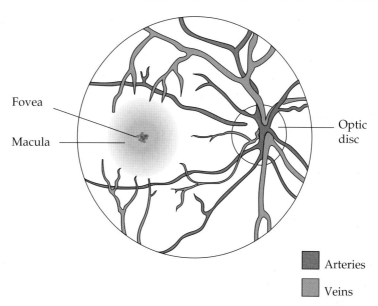

Fovea

Macula

Optic disc

Arteries

Veins

FIGURE 1.18 Fundus diagram.

and typically have a more prominent light reflex than veins. The examiner should follow arteries from the disc and veins back to the disc in each quadrant, noting in particular the arteriovenous (A/V) crossing patterns.

Fundus Background

The normal fundus background is a uniform red-orange color primarily due to the pigmentation of the retinal pigment epithelium. The blood and pigment of the choroid also contribute to the appearance of the fundus background. For example, in heavily pigmented eyes, the fundus may have a darker color due to increased choroidal pigment content.

Fovea

The normal fovea, at the center of the macula (see Figures 1.15 and 1.18), is located directly temporal and slightly inferior to the optic disc and usually appears darker than the surrounding retina because the specialized retinal pigment epithelial cells of the fovea are taller and more heavily pigmented. In some eyes, the fovea may appear slightly yellow due to the xanthophyll pigment in the retina. The central depression of the fovea may act as a concave mirror during ophthalmoscopy and produce a light reflection known as the *foveal reflex.*

SUMMARY OF STEPS IN EYE EXAMINATION

An accurate history must be obtained before beginning the physical examination.

1. Measure the visual acuity for each eye.
2. Perform a confrontation field test for each eye.

3. Inspect the lids and the surrounding tissues.
4. Inspect the conjunctiva and sclera.
5. Test the extraocular movements.
6. Test the pupils for direct and consensual responses.
7. Inspect the cornea and iris.
8. Assess the anterior chamber for depth and clarity.
9. Assess the lens for clarity through direct ophthalmoscopy.
10. Use the ophthalmoscope to study the fundus, including the disc, vessels, and macula.
11. Perform tonometry when acute angle-closure glaucoma is suspected, if a reliable tonometer is available.

MANAGEMENT OR REFERRAL

The American Academy of Ophthalmology recommends that patients ages 40 to 65 be examined by an ophthalmologist every 2 to 4 years (after receiving a baseline exam at age 40 if not previously done), and every 1 to 2 years for patients over age 65. Children should undergo an evaluation in the first few months of life, then again at 6 months, 3 years, and 5 years of age by their primary care physician. Any abnormalities should be evaluated by an ophthalmologist (see Chapter 6).

REDUCED VISUAL ACUITY

The following guidelines apply for patients in whom reduced visual acuity is found, unless the patient has been seen by an ophthalmologist and the condition has been confirmed as stable.

VA Less Than 20/20

Any patient with visual acuity less than 20/20 in 1 or both eyes should be referred to an ophthalmologist if visual symptoms are present. Reduced visual acuity is the best single criterion by which to differentiate potentially blinding conditions from less serious ocular disorders, although 20/20 visual acuity does not preclude a patient from having serious eye disease.

VA Less Than 20/40

Any patient with visual acuity less than 20/40 in both eyes is an equally important candidate for referral, even in the absence of complaints. Although many such patients suffer only from uncorrected refractive errors, undetected painless but progressive loss of vision does occur in many disorders of the eyes and visual system.

Asymmetry

Any patient with a difference in visual acuity between the eyes of 2 lines or more on the Snellen chart should be referred promptly, even if visual acuity in 1 or both eyes is better than 20/40. Generally, visual function is nearly identical between the eyes; thus, in the absence of known causes of reduced vision, asymmetry of visual acuity may be a sign of occult disease. Patients may be unaware of even severe vision loss in 1 eye if the other eye sees normally.

Presbyopia

Presbyopia is manifested by reduced near vision with no change in distance visual acuity. Middle-aged or elderly patients complaining of this combination will benefit from a referral for the prescription of corrective lenses.

ABNORMAL FUNDUS APPEARANCE

Only after performing numerous fundus examinations will the practitioner be able to recognize the great range of normal ophthalmoscopic appearances. When an abnormality is suspected, further studies or consultation may be required because fundus abnormalities can indicate significant ocular or systemic diseases. Ophthalmologic consultation should be sought for fundus changes accompanied by acute or chronic visual complaints or in patients with systemic disease known to manifest in the eye (see Chapter 8).

Photographs of the fundus are taken with a special camera that provides a greater field of view than is possible with the direct ophthalmoscope. Many fundus abnormalities have 3-dimensional qualities, such as elevation or depression, but the examiner is limited to a monocular, 2-dimensional view with the direct ophthalmoscope or photographs. It is necessary to learn to think in 3 dimensions in order to grasp the pathophysiology.

SHALLOW ANTERIOR CHAMBER DEPTH/ELEVATED INTRAOCULAR PRESSURE

A patient suspected of having shallow anterior chamber depth (at risk for angle-closure glaucoma) should be referred to an ophthalmologist for further evaluation.

POINTS TO REMEMBER

- An inadequate history can lead the physician to misinterpret the examination findings.
- To prevent patients from reading the visual acuity chart with both eyes, either intentionally or unintentionally, the examiner must ensure that 1 eye is completely occluded.
- A well-lighted hallway often provides an acceptable location for distance visual acuity testing with a standard Snellen chart.
- To avoid measurement error when performing tonometry, the examiner must keep the lids apart by holding them firmly against the bony margins of the orbit, rather than by pressing them against the globe.

SAMPLE PROBLEMS

1. A 14-year-old boy is seen for a physical examination at school. He admits to difficulty in seeing details across the classroom, but not in reading textbooks. He does not wear glasses. You record VA as OD 20/100, pinhole 20/25; and OS

20/100, pinhole 20/25. What is your diagnosis? Would you manage or refer this patient?

Answer: The combination of decreased distance vision with preserved near vision is typical of myopia, which often becomes symptomatic during adolescence. Presumptive evidence of refractive error is provided by the marked improvement in visual acuity that occurs with the use of the pinhole. Note that visual acuity with use of the pinhole frequently does not reach 20/20. The patient should be referred to an ophthalmologist as a regular rather than an urgent consultation.

2. A 78-year-old woman is seen for an annual physical examination and complains of mild difficulty in reading and in seeing street signs. You record OD 20/70, no improvement with pinhole; and OS 20/50, no improvement with pinhole. Upon direct ophthalmoscopy, you note a dullness of the red reflex and you have difficulty seeing fundus details in both eyes. What is your diagnosis? Would you manage or refer this patient?

Answer: Cataract is a common cause of painless progressive loss of vision in older individuals. Her complaints about her visual ability are an indication for referral to an ophthalmologist for evaluation for possible cataract surgery.

3. A 40-year-old man is seen for an annual executive physical. He has no complaints and does not wear glasses. You record VA as OD 20/15 and OS 20/100, no improvement with pinhole. During examination, the patient revealed that he has been aware since childhood that his left eye is a so-called lazy eye—in other words, that he suffered from amblyopia. Would you refer this patient?

Answer: Referral is not indicated since the cause of decreased vision is established and progressive loss is not occurring. However, it is important to emphasize wearing appropriate eye protection during home and outdoor activities that would put his better eye at risk of injury.

4. A 50-year-old man visits your office because he noted decreased visual acuity in the right eye the preceding day while accidentally occluding his left eye. When his present glasses were prescribed 2 years ago, his vision was equal in both eyes. You record VA as OD 20/50, no improvement with pinhole; and OS 20/20. Upon ophthalmoscopy, no abnormalities are detected. What, if any, is your diagnosis? Would you manage or refer this patient?

Answer: The patient has an unexplained loss of vision of unknown duration in 1 eye. An unexplained decrease in vision in 1 or both eyes requires referral to an ophthalmologist, because it may indicate occult disease of the eyes or central nervous system that is not detectable by examination methods available to the primary care physician. In this case, the patient's decreased vision was due to a macular disturbance detectable only by more precise methods of examination (eg, special lenses and fluorescein angiography).

5. A 55-year-old man, wearing safety goggles, was sawing wood in his garage shop. He removed the goggles to clean up and, while sweeping up small wood chips, had the sudden onset of a foreign-body sensation in his right eye. The irritation was not relieved with artificial tears, and it intensified with every blink. His wife rushed him to their family doctor for emergency treatment. The physician was able to examine him after placing a topical anesthetic in the right eye. Visual acuity in the right eye was 20/80. Fluorescein staining revealed multiple vertical linear abrasions of the cornea.

    A. Explain the clinical findings.

    Answer: By history, this man has been exposed to small particles that could abrade his eye. The vertical linear abrasions in conjunction with the feeling of irritation with each blink imply the presence of a foreign body under the upper lid.

    B. What further examination is required, and how is it performed?

    Answer: Eversion of the upper lid (see Figure 1.9) will expose the foreign body, which can then be removed using a cotton-tipped applicator stick.

6. A 64-year-old woman visits your office complaining of flashing lights in her peripheral vision. You obtain the following details in your history of present illness. In her right eye only, the lights have been present for several days. Numerous small, dark floaters accompany them. On the day of presentation, she began to note a dark area in the superotemporal visual field of the affected eye. Her visual acuity is 20/20 in each eye, and your physical exam of the patient through undilated pupils is unremarkable. What is your diagnosis?

    a. Ocular migraine
    b. Branch retinal artery occlusion
    c. Retinal detachment
    d. Refractive error

    Answer: c. This patient's symptoms are very suspicious for a retinal detachment, and she should be examined by an ophthalmologist urgently. The history is key in making the diagnosis. The duration, location (unilateral versus bilateral), and associated symptoms all are compatible with a retinal tear or retinal detachment. Prompt referral is indicated despite the lack of physical findings because the peripheral retina is not readily examined with a direct ophthalmoscope.

ANNOTATED RESOURCES

Chou R, Dana T, Bougatsos C. Screening older adults for impaired visual acuity: a review of the evidence for the U.S. Preventive Services Task Force. *Ann Intern Med.* 2009;151:44–58, W11-20.

Doughty MJ, Laiquzzaman M, Button NF. Video-assessment of tear meniscus height in elderly Caucasians and its relationship to the exposed ocular surface. *Curr Eye Res.* 2001;22:420–426.

Gayton JL. Etiology, prevalence, and treatment of dry eye disease. *Clin Ophthalmol.* 2009;3:405–412.

Gittinger JW Jr. *Ophthalmology: A Clinical Introduction.* Boston, MA: Little, Brown & Co; 1984. Chapter 1, "Ocular History and Examination," covers the eye examination in this excellent introductory text for medical students.

Jackson GR, Owsley C, McGwin G Jr. Aging and dark adaptation. *Vision Res.* 1999;39:3975–3982.

Kim JS, Sharpe JA. The vertical vestibulo-ocular reflex, and its interaction with vision during active head motion: effects of aging. *J Vestib Res.* 2001;11:3–12.

Movaghar MD, Lawrence MG. "Eye Exam: The Essentials." In: *The Eye Examination and Ophthalmic Instruments.* San Francisco, CA: American Academy of Ophthalmology; 2001, reviewed for currency in 2007. Three titles on the DVD provide the basic framework for the ocular examination of an adult or child, as well as the use of common ophthalmic instruments.

Newell FW. *Ophthalmology: Principles and Concepts.* 8th ed. St Louis, MO: CV Mosby Co; 1996. This comprehensive text covers in detail anatomy (Chapter 1), physiology (Chapter 2), symptoms of eye disease (Chapter 4), and examination techniques (Chapters 5 and 6).

Nomura H, Tanabe N, Hagaya S, et al. Eye examinations at the National Institute for Longevity Sciences—Longitudinal Study of Aging: NILS-LSA. *J Epidemiol.* 2000;10(1 Suppl): S18–S25.

Pavan-Langston D, ed. *Manual of Ocular Diagnosis and Therapy.* 5th ed. Philadelphia, PA: Lippincott Williams & Wilkins; 2002. Chapter 1, "Ocular Examination Techniques and Diagnostic Tests," covers the full gamut of techniques, including those that would be used only by an ophthalmologist.

Trobe JD. *The Physician's Guide to Eye Care.* 3rd ed. San Francisco, CA: American Academy of Ophthalmology; 2006. This brief but comprehensive and well-illustrated resource covers the principal clinical ophthalmic problems that nonophthalmologist physicians are likely to encounter, organized for practical use by practitioners. Chapter 1 presents techniques for performing a screening examination, and Chapter 2 outlines rationale, frequency, and components of the routine examination for asymptomatic patients.

Vaughan DG, Asbury T, Riordan-Eva P, eds. *General Ophthalmology*. 17th ed. Norwalk, CT: Appleton & Lange; 2007. This is a useful and popular textbook for medical students, ophthalmology residents, and other physicians. Chapter 1, "Anatomy & Embryology of the Eye," contains good anatomic illustrations; Chapter 2, "Ophthalmologic Examination," contains information on ophthalmic instruments and examination techniques.

Wilson FM II, ed. *Practical Ophthalmology: A Manual for Beginning Ophthalmology Residents*. 6th ed. San Francisco, CA: American Academy of Ophthalmology; 2009. Intended for beginning ophthalmology residents, this comprehensive book presents numerous step-by-step protocols for a wide range of basic ophthalmologic examinations, which medical students and residents may find useful.

Acute Visual Loss

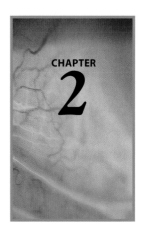

OBJECTIVES

As a primary care physician, you should be able to evaluate a patient complaining of a sudden decrease in visual acuity or visual field, to construct a differential diagnosis, and to recognize situations requiring urgent action. To achieve these objectives, you should learn

- ➤ Which questions to ask the patient
- ➤ Which examination techniques are appropriate, with special attention to pupillary responses, visual field testing, and ophthalmoscopy
- ➤ Which conditions are most likely to cause acute visual loss

RELEVANCE

For most people, sudden visual loss is a devastating occurrence. The primary care physician needs to recognize the conditions responsible for acute visual loss in order to make urgent referrals to an ophthalmologist and to actually initiate therapy, when appropriate. The ultimate visual outcome may well depend on early, accurate diagnosis and timely treatment.

BASIC INFORMATION

Obtaining the patient's history is vitally important in determining the cause of acute vision loss. The value of a thorough history cannot be overstated; although the physical examination provides necessary information, often the history itself guides the clinician to the correct diagnosis. Questions to ask the patient in the wake of sudden visual loss include

- What is the patient's age and medical condition?
- Is the visual loss transient, persistent, or progressive?
- Is the visual loss monocular or binocular?
- How severe is the loss of vision?

- What was the tempo? Did the visual loss occur abruptly, or did it develop over hours, days, or weeks?
- Did the patient have normal vision (with glasses if needed) in the past?
- Was pain associated with the visual loss?

HOW TO EXAMINE

The following examination techniques aid in your evaluation of visual loss.

VISUAL ACUITY TESTING

The first thing to be determined in evaluating acute visual loss is the visual acuity, with best available correction, in each eye. (For detailed information on visual acuity testing, see Chapter 1.)

CONFRONTATION VISUAL FIELD TESTING

Normal acuity does not assure that significant vision has not been lost, because the entire visual field, including peripheral vision, must be considered. For instance, a patient who has lost all of the peripheral vision on 1 side in both eyes—a homonymous hemianopia—may have normal visual acuity. For instruction on assessing the visual field through confrontation visual field testing (see Chapter 1).

PUPILLARY REACTIONS

The reaction of the pupils to light is useful in the evaluation of visual loss, especially when that reaction is asymmetric. In the swinging-flashlight test, a bright light is moved from one eye to the other and the pupillary reactions are observed. When there is a significant lesion in the retina or the optic nerve of one eye, the brainstem centers controlling pupillary size perceive the light as being brighter in the normal eye. Thus, when the light beam is moved from the normal eye to the abnormal eye, the pupil of the abnormal eye may continue to dilate. This positive swinging-flashlight test indicates a relative afferent pupillary defect, also known as a *Marcus Gunn* pupil. The presence or absence of a relative afferent pupillary defect is an important piece of information in the evaluation of monocular visual loss. (For more information on pupillary reactions and the swinging-flashlight test, see Chapter 7.)

OPHTHALMOSCOPY

Ophthalmoscopy is probably the most important examination technique in the evaluation of visual loss because it allows direct inspection of the fundus and an assessment of the clarity of the refractive media, the red reflex. (For information on the technique of direct ophthalmoscopy, see Chapter 1.)

PENLIGHT EXAMINATION

Simple penlight examination may detect corneal disease responsible for acute visual loss.

TONOMETRY

Tonometry to measure intraocular pressure (IOP) may help confirm the presence of angle-closure glaucoma. (For more information about performing tonometry, see Chapter 1.)

HOW TO INTERPRET THE FINDINGS

The following conditions are often implicated in cases of visual loss.

MEDIA OPACITIES

Any significant irregularity or opacity of the clear refractive media of the eye (cornea, anterior chamber, lens, vitreous) causes symptoms of blurred vision, and on examination there is a reduction of visual acuity and a darkening of the red reflex. These opacities do not cause relative afferent pupillary defects, although pupillary reflexes may be altered (eg, miosis in acute iritis or mid-dilated and fixed pupils in acute angle-closure glaucoma). Acute visual loss may result from conditions that cause rapid changes in the transparency of these tissues.

CORNEAL EDEMA

One cause of sudden opacification of the cornea is corneal edema, which is recognized by a dulling of the normally crisp reflection of incident light off the cornea. The cornea, crystal-clear when healthy, takes on a ground-glass appearance.

A common cause of corneal edema is increased IOP. Visual loss accompanying an attack of angle-closure glaucoma (an ocular emergency) is largely the result of corneal edema (see Figure 4.10). Corneal endothelial cell dysfunction due to dystrophies, or sometimes following intraocular surgery, can result in corneal edema, but the visual loss generally has a gradual onset. Any acute infection or inflammation of the cornea (eg, herpes simplex keratitis) may mimic corneal edema.

HYPHEMA

Blood in the anterior chamber is known as a *hyphema* (see Figure 5.3). Any significant hyphema reduces vision, and a complete hyphema will reduce vision to light perception only. Lesser degrees of hyphema may not affect visual acuity. Most hyphemas are the direct consequence of blunt trauma to a normal eye; however, the presence of abnormal iris vessels (which occurs with tumors, diabetes, intraocular surgery, and chronic inflammation—all causes of neovascularization) predisposes the patient to hyphema, which may be spontaneous (not associated with trauma).

CATARACT

Most cataracts develop slowly. The rare patient may interpret rapid progression of a cataract as sudden visual loss. Even in a patient with a clear lens, sudden changes in blood sugar or serum electrolytes can alter the hydration of the lens. These changes in lens hydration can result in large fluctuations in refractive error, which may be interpreted by the patient as visual loss. In this situation, acuity may simply be improved with refraction.

VITREOUS HEMORRHAGE

Bleeding into the vitreous (Figure 2.1) reduces vision in the same way that hyphema does: in relation to the amount and location of opaque blood. Large vitreous hemorrhages may occur after trauma and in any condition causing retinal neovascularization (eg, proliferative diabetic retinopathy, retinal vein occlusion, or proliferative sickle cell retinopathy). Retinal tears may present with a vitreous hemorrhage. In addition, vitreous hemorrhage may accompany subarachnoid hemorrhage and is one cause of visual loss from intracranial aneurysms. Vitreous hemorrhage may be difficult to appreciate when viewed with the ophthalmoscope, especially through an undilated pupil. If the red reflex cannot be seen but the lens appears clear, vitreous hemorrhage should be suspected. Diagnosis can be confirmed by an ophthalmologist with slit-lamp examination through a dilated pupil.

RETINAL DISEASE

Retinal detachment, macular disease, and retinal vascular occlusion are all associated with sudden visual loss. Acute visual loss may develop in any inflammatory process that affects the retina, including infectious chorioretinitis, vasculitides, and idiopathic inflammation. These conditions may be distinguished from other causes of acute visual loss by their ophthalmoscopic findings.

Retinal Detachment

Acute visual loss is a feature of an extensive retinal detachment. Typically, the patient with a retinal detachment (Figure 2.2) complains of flashing lights, called *photopsia*, followed by large numbers of floaters and then a shade over the vision in 1 eye. A detachment extensive enough to reduce visual acuity may produce a relative afferent pupillary defect in the involved eye. The diagnosis of an extensive

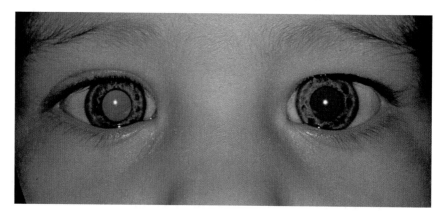

FIGURE 2.1 Vitreous hemorrhage seen in red reflex. Ophthalmoscopic examination reveals a darkened red reflex from the patient's left eye resulting from a vitreous hemorrhage. (Courtesy WK Kellogg Eye Center, University of Michigan)

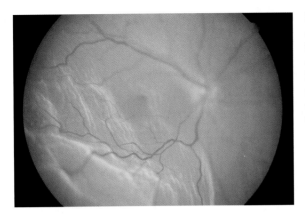

FIGURE 2.2 Retinal detachment. A wide-angle photograph of the fundus reveals folds of retina extending into the macula inferotemporal to the disc. In this photograph, the focus is on the elevated retina, which renders the disc slightly out of focus.

retinal detachment is made by ophthalmoscopy through the dilated pupil. The retina appears elevated, sometimes with folds, and the choroidal background is indistinct. However, the findings may not be obvious, and emergency ophthalmologic consultation is indicated if retinal detachment is suspected.

Macular Disease

Macular disease reduces visual acuity, but unless the disease is extensive, a relative afferent pupillary defect may not be present. Sudden visual loss or metamorphopsia (a defect of central vision in which the shapes of objects appear distorted) from macular disease is often a sign of bleeding from a neovascular net formed as part of the process of age-related macular degeneration (see Chapter 3). If neovascularization is identified it may be treated with an injection of a medication that causes inhibition and regression of the pathological vessels, or with laser surgery.

Retinal Vascular Occlusion

Retinal vascular occlusion is a relatively common cause of sudden visual loss and may be transient or permanent. Transient monocular visual loss due to arterial insufficiency is called *amaurosis fugax* and is a very important symptom. In a patient over age 50, the report of visual loss in 1 eye lasting for several minutes should lead to investigation of the ipsilateral carotid circulation, looking for an atheroma. The valves and chambers of the heart should also be investigated, looking for an embolic source causing transient interruption of blood flow to the retina (Figure 2.3). The evaluation and management of such a patient raises complicated issues, and referral should be made to an ophthalmologist, a neurologist, or a vascular surgeon, depending on the results of the workup.

Central Retinal Artery Occlusion

Prolonged interruption of retinal arterial blood flow causes permanent damage to the ganglion cells and other tissue elements. Central retinal artery occlusion (CRAO, Figure 2.4) is manifested as a sudden, painless, and often severe visual

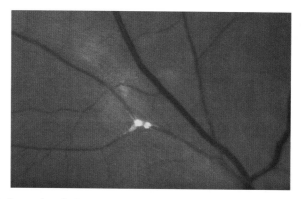

FIGURE 2.3 Cholesterol embolus in retinal arteriole. In the elderly, the most common sources of emboli are fibrin and cholesterol from ulcerated plaques in the wall of the carotid artery. The so-called *Hollenhorst plaque* is a cholesterol embolus that lodges at an arterial bifurcation, as shown here. (Reprinted from "Ocular Manifestations of Systemic Disease." In: *Eye Care Skills: Presentations for Physicians and Other Health Care Professionals,* v3.0. San Francisco: American Academy of Ophthalmology; 2009.)

loss. The ophthalmoscopic appearance depends on how soon after the visual loss the fundus is seen. Within minutes to hours, the only findings may be vascular stasis: narrowing of arterial blood columns and interruption of venous blood columns with the appearance of "boxcarring" as rows of corpuscles are separated by clear intervals.

Some hours after a CRAO, the inner layer of the retina becomes opalescent. The loss of the normal transparency of the retina is most visible ophthalmoscopically where the retina is thickest around the fovea. In the fovea itself, the inner layers are attenuated and the underlying intact choroidal circulation is seen. Pallor of the perifoveal retina stands in contrast to the normal color of the fovea, causing the characteristic "cherry-red spot" of CRAO. (A chronic cherry-red spot is also a feature of storage diseases, such as Tay-Sachs disease and some variants of Niemann-Pick disease, in which the ganglion cells become opalescent because of the deposition of intermediate metabolites.)

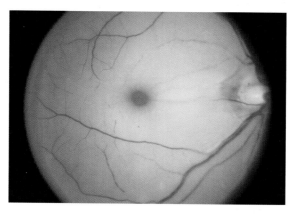

FIGURE 2.4 Central retinal artery occlusion. The retina is opaque, except for the relatively thin area within the macula, producing the "cherry-red spot."

The optic disc, which is supplied by other branches of the ophthalmic artery, does not swell unless the occlusion is in the ophthalmic or carotid artery, proximal to the origin of the central retinal artery or in the small vessels supplying the disc. The peculiarities of the eye's vascular supply also can explain the possible preservation of some vision in the presence of a complete CRAO. If part of the retina derives its blood supply from the choroidal circulation via a cilioretinal artery, its function is spared. After a CRAO, the retinal edema slowly resolves, and the death of the ganglion cells and their axons leads to optic atrophy. Months later, the characteristic ophthalmoscopic appearance is a pale disc in a blind eye.

When ophthalmoscopy reveals an acute CRAO, immediate treatment is warranted unless circulation has already been restored spontaneously. *This is a true ophthalmic emergency*; restoration of blood flow may preserve vision if the occlusion is only a few hours old. Instances have been reported in which vision returned after treatment of an occlusion that had been present for several days. In a blind eye, there is little to lose by aggressive measures, and an ophthalmologist's advice should be obtained emergently.

As an emergency measure, the primary care physician may wish to compress the eye with the heel of the hand, pressing firmly for 10 seconds and then releasing for 10 seconds over a period of approximately 5 minutes. The sudden rise and fall in intraocular pressure could serve to dislodge a small embolus in the central retinal artery and restore circulation before the retinal tissues sustain irreversible damage. An ophthalmologist might employ more vigorous and invasive techniques, such as medications to lower IOP, vasodilators, and paracentesis of the anterior chamber. Although most retinal artery occlusions are embolic in nature, central or branch retinal artery occlusion in an elderly patient without a visible embolus should be evaluated for giant cell arteritis.

Branch Retinal Artery Occlusion

When only a branch of the central retinal artery is occluded, only a sector of the retina opacifies, producing only a partial loss of vision. The patient will often know the moment of vision loss and may be able to describe or draw the exact outline of the missing area of vision. A branch retinal artery occlusion (BRAO, Figure 2.5) is

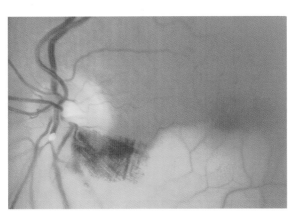

FIGURE 2.5 Branch retinal artery occlusion. Inferotemporal branch retinal artery obstruction. (Courtesy Cynthia A. Bradford, MD)

more likely to be the result of an embolus than is a CRAO, and a source should be sought. If visual acuity is affected, attempts should be made to dislodge the embolus by ocular massage, as discussed above.

Central Retinal Vein Occlusion

The ophthalmoscopic picture of disc swelling, venous engorgement, cotton-wool spots (which appear as small white patches on the retina), and diffuse retinal hemorrhages indicates a central retinal vein occlusion (CRVO, Figure 2.6). Visual loss may be severe, although the onset is generally subacute, unlike the dramatic sudden blindness of CRAO. The fundus picture can be so striking that the description "blood and thunder" is applied. Despite its dramatic appearance, there is no generally accepted acute management, and a CRVO is not a true ophthalmic emergency.

A CRVO is most often encountered in older patients with hypertension and arteriosclerotic vascular disease. Carotid artery occlusion may produce a similar but milder fundus picture. In rare cases, diseases that increase blood viscosity—such as polycythemia vera, sickle-cell disease, and lymphoma-leukemia—induce a CRVO.

The acute hemorrhages and disc swelling resolve with time; however, they may be followed by the development of shunt vessels from the retinal to the choroidal circulation or by ocular neovascularization. The patient with a CRVO needs a general medical evaluation and follow-up by an ophthalmologist, who may be able to prevent the late complication of neovascular glaucoma in susceptible patients by performing laser photocoagulation surgery of the ischemic retina.

OPTIC NERVE DISEASE

Conditions affecting the optic nerve can often result in acute visual loss. Although the optic nerve head may or may not appear normal initially by ophthalmoscopy, pupillary responses are usually abnormal in unilateral disease.

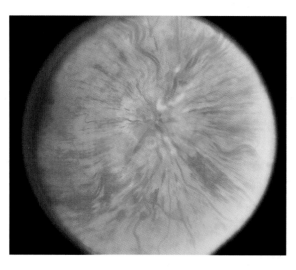

FIGURE 2.6 Central retinal vein occlusion. Dilated and tortuous veins, flame-shaped hemorrhages, and cotton-wool spots characterize this condition. Sometimes this is referred to as a "blood and thunder" retinal appearance.

Optic Neuritis

Optic neuritis is an inflammation of the optic nerve that is usually idiopathic but may be associated with multiple sclerosis in a significant number of cases. Reduced visual acuity and a relative afferent pupillary defect are regular features of optic neuritis. The patient may complain that colors appear desaturated or washed out and that things appear darker when viewed with the affected eye. The optic disc appears hyperemic and swollen (the disc margin is blurred and no discrete edge can be discerned). The prognosis for the return of vision after a single attack of optic neuritis is good. Patients with suspected optic neuritis should be referred to an ophthalmologist for further evaluation. Certain patients with optic neuritis may benefit from high-dose intravenous corticosteroids (oral corticosteroids are contraindicated).

Retrobulbar Optic Neuritis

A young adult who is experiencing a monocular, stepwise, progressive loss of vision that has developed over hours to days and that is often accompanied by pain on movement of the eye but who shows no abnormalities on ophthalmoscopic examination probably has retrobulbar optic neuritis. Again, vision is usually poor and an afferent pupillary defect is present. Included in the differential diagnosis of retrobulbar optic neuritis is *compressive optic neuropathy*, which can appear as acute visual loss. The pattern of visual field loss may point to a noninflammatory cause, for example, by a finding of visual field loss in the other eye. Computed tomography or magnetic resonance imaging of the orbits and chiasmal region will identify most compressive lesions, which are potentially treatable with surgery.

Papillitis and Papilledema

Like retrobulbar optic neuritis, papillitis (Figure 2.7) is a subtype of optic neuritis. Specifically, *papillitis* is an inflammation of the optic disc, or papilla. *Papilledema* (Figure 2.8), on the other hand, refers to swelling of the optic disc from increased intracranial pressure; both optic discs are affected. In optic neuritis (either

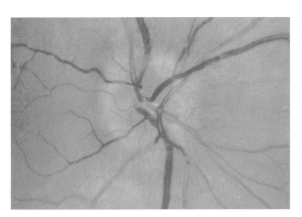

FIGURE 2.7 Papillitis. The disc is swollen, with blurred disc margins. In papillitis, the disc is hyperemic, rather than pale as in ischemic optic neuropathy. Papillitis is usually unilateral. Bilateral papillitis can be differentiated from papilledema based on decreased visual acuity in papillitis.

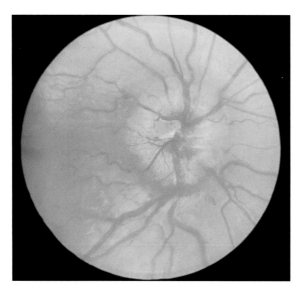

FIGURE 2.8 Papilledema. The optic disc is elevated and the margins are indistinct. There is microvascular congestion on the disc, the retinal veins are dilated, and flame-shaped hemorrhages are present. The appearance in the other eye should be similar.

retrobulbar neuritis or papillitis), vision is usually (but not always) significantly decreased, and examination of the pupils will reveal a relative afferent pupillary defect. In papilledema, the visual acuity and the pupillary reflexes are usually normal. In both conditions, fundus examination will reveal blurred optic disc margins, and the optic disc cupping is typically obliterated.

Some patients with acute papilledema complain of momentary blurring or transient obscurations of vision. Although chronic papilledema may lead to loss of vision, most patients with acute papilledema suffer only minor alterations in vision. An emergent brain scan to identify an intracranial mass is indicated. Patients with pseudotumor cerebri will have papilledema without a midline shift on brain scan, and a spinal tap is necessary to document increased intracranial pressure.

Ischemic Optic Neuropathy

Swelling of the disc accompanied by visual loss in an older adult is likely to represent a vascular event rather than inflammation. *Ischemic optic neuropathy* (Figure 2.9) is a vascular disorder that presents as a pale, swollen disc, often accompanied by splinter hemorrhages and loss of visual acuity and visual field. The field loss with ischemic neuropathy is often predominantly in the superior or inferior field, a pattern known as *altitudinal*.

Giant Cell Arteritis

The development of acute ischemic optic neuropathy in a patient over age 60 raises the possibility of giant cell, or temporal, arteritis. Patients being considered for the diagnosis of giant cell arteritis (GCA) should undergo a focused review of systems. Common complaints associated with GCA are temporal headache or tenderness, often causing pain while resting on a pillow; scalp tenderness with hair brushing;

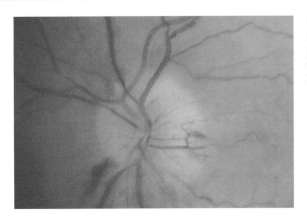

FIGURE 2.9 Ischemic optic neuropathy. This figure shows pale swelling of the optic disc, with associated flame-shaped hemorrhages.

ear or anterior neck discomfort (carotidynia); fatigue or pain in the tongue or jaw with chewing (jaw claudication); and episodes of transient diplopia or visual loss. Other complaints include anorexia, weight loss, general malaise, and aching/fatigue of the upper arms or legs (polymyalgia rheumatica).

Even in an otherwise asymptomatic elderly patient who has ischemic optic neuropathy (or, for that matter, a CRAO or an unexplained ophthalmoplegia, a paresis of extraocular movement), an erythrocyte sedimentation rate and a C-reactive protein level should be obtained immediately. Many elderly persons with GCA have markedly elevated sedimentation rates, to greater than 60 mm per hour. If the sedimentation rate is elevated or if there are other symptoms or signs of GCA, treatment with high-dose systemic corticosteroids is mandatory unless there is a very strong contraindication to their use. This course of treatment may preserve vision in the remaining eye and prevent vascular occlusions elsewhere that would cause stroke or myocardial infarction. *Immediate referral to an ophthalmologist is indicated if giant cell arteritis is a strong diagnostic possibility.* Biopsy of the temporal artery may demonstrate pathologic changes that confirm the diagnosis: giant cells, fragmentation of the elastica with surrounding chronic inflammation, and, sometimes, occlusion of the vessel.

If no systemic arteritis is demonstrated, there is no clear evidence that systemic corticosteroids benefit patients with ischemic optic neuropathy. Unfortunately, there is an approximately 40% chance that the other eye will become involved with nonarteritic ischemic optic neuropathy, with or without treatment.

Trauma

Trauma is another potential cause of visual loss due to involvement of the optic nerve (traumatic optic neuropathy). Visual loss may be mild to severe and may recover spontaneously. In a small number of cases, concussive head trauma shears the vascular supply to the optic nerve, producing blindness. Treatment with high-dose intravenous corticosteroids or surgical decompression of the optic canal may be undertaken in selected cases.

VISUAL PATHWAY DISORDERS

The following disorders should be considered in occurrences of acute visual loss.

Hemianopia

The cerebral visual pathways are susceptible to involvement by vascular events or tumors. In older persons, a *homonymous* hemianopia, defined as loss of vision on 1 side of both visual fields, may result from occlusion of 1 of the posterior cerebral arteries with infarction of the occipital lobe. Other vascular events occurring in the middle cerebral artery distribution also may produce a hemianopia, but usually other neurologic signs are prominent. Almost any patient with a hemianopia warrants examination by cerebral computed tomography or magnetic resonance imaging to localize and identify the cause. (See Chapter 7 for more information about hemianopic visual field loss.)

Cortical Blindness

Much rarer than a hemianopia is extensive bilateral damage to the cerebral visual pathways resulting in complete loss of vision. This condition is referred to variously as *cortical, central,* or *cerebral blindness.* Because the pathways serving the pupillary light reflex separate from those carrying visual information at the level of the optic tracts, a patient who is cortically blind has normal pupillary reactions. This finding, along with a normal fundus on ophthalmoscopic examination, helps make the diagnosis of cortical blindness. Transient cortical blindness has been observed in children after concussive head trauma.

FUNCTIONAL DISORDERS

The adjective *functional* is used in preference to *hysterical* or *malingering* to describe visual loss without organic basis. Often the diagnosis is apparent because the examination produces results incompatible with organic blindness. For example, the patient who reports complete blindness in one eye and normal vision in the other but has normal stereopsis and no relative afferent pupillary defect most likely has a functional disorder. In other patients, sophisticated ophthalmologic examinations may be necessary to make an accurate diagnosis.

ACUTE DISCOVERY OF CHRONIC VISUAL LOSS

A surprising number of cases of chronic visual loss turn up as acute discoveries. Because the eyes usually function together, this sudden discovery of what has actually been an ongoing problem is most likely to occur when the vision in 1 eye is normal. A person who claims acute visual loss in 1 eye but has advanced optic atrophy must have had a prolonged but unrecognized problem. In doubtful cases, it is desirable to obtain records of previous formal eye examinations before accepting visual loss as an acute event and proceeding with expensive or invasive workups.

POINTS TO REMEMBER

- Early, accurate diagnosis and timely treatment are critical to a positive visual outcome in cases of acute visual loss.
- Patient ocular history, including timing, tempo, and unilaterality or bilaterality of visual loss, as well as medical history and prior visual acuity, are important to making an accurate diagnosis.
- Pupillary responses, visual field testing, and ophthalmoscopy to evaluate the red reflex as well as the fundus are particularly valuable in determining the causes of acute visual loss.
- The following conditions require emergency measures and referral: retinal detachment, acute central retinal artery occlusion, and ischemic optic neuropathy if suspected to be related to giant cell arteritis.

SAMPLE PROBLEMS

1. A 70-year-old man notes sudden profound loss of vision in his right eye, with onset 2 hours ago. The vision loss has not changed since the onset. The patient has a past medical history of hypertension. On examination, the visual acuity is OD hand motion and OS 20/20. The right pupil does not respond to light directly but does react consensually. The left pupil reacts to light directly but not consensually. The swinging-flashlight test confirms a right relative afferent pupillary defect (Marcus Gunn pupil). The direct ophthalmoscope shows that the red reflex is clear in both eyes. Retinal examination reveals a white, opacified retina with a cherry-red macular spot. The left retina is normal. You diagnose a central retinal artery occlusion. What is the proper management?

   Answer: You apply pressure to the patient's right eye by placing the heel of your hand on the patient's closed eyelid and pressing and releasing several times. The goal of this ocular massage is to dislodge a retinal embolus. Lowering the IOP using intravenous acetazolamide or topical glaucoma drops may also help dislodge the embolus. Immediate ophthalmologic consultation is indicated. The patient should be evaluated for the cause of this retinal vascular event. Because the retina is neural tissue and survives complete circulatory deprivation poorly, the prognosis for recovery of useful vision in the affected eye is guarded. It is important to detect underlying disease or a site of embolus formation (such as carotid atheroma or cardiac valvular disease) that might lead to future vascular occlusions.

2. A 24-year-old woman notes sudden visual loss in her left eye. She is in otherwise good health. On examination, her visual acuity is OD 20/20, OS 20/100. Examination of the pupillary light reflexes with the swinging-flashlight test reveals a relative afferent pupillary defect OS. The anterior segment examination is normal. The red reflex is clear in both eyes. The retinal examination is

normal in the right eye but reveals a swollen optic disc in the left eye. What is your course of action?

Answer: The findings of sudden reduced acuity, clear ocular media, a relative afferent pupillary defect, and a swollen optic disc in a healthy young woman suggest a diagnosis of optic neuritis. Consultation with a neurologist and an ophthalmologist or a neuro-ophthalmologist is indicated. After a neurologic assessment, the patient may need additional testing such as magnetic resonance imaging and assessment of cerebrospinal fluid. In some cases, treatment with intravenous corticosteroids is indicated. The majority of patients with optic neuritis can expect improvement in their vision. Some patients with optic neuritis develop multiple sclerosis.

3. A 90-year-old woman has recently noticed visual loss OD, along with a persistent right-sided headache, generalized fatigue, and a 10-pound weight loss. Your examination reveals a visual acuity of OD 20/80 and OS 20/30. There is a right relative afferent pupillary defect. Confrontation visual field assessment shows inferior visual field loss in the right eye; the left eye is normal. On dilated retinal examination, the right optic disc is swollen and there are flame-shaped hemorrhages around the disc. What is your course of action?

Answer: Your index of suspicion should be high for giant cell arteritis in this elderly patient due to the sudden vision loss, afferent pupillary defect, swollen disc, weight loss, and headache. You should obtain stat erythrocyte sedimentation rate and C-reactive protein tests and refer the patient to an ophthalmologist immediately. The patient will need high-dose corticosteroid treatment to preserve vision in the fellow eye and prevent other systemic complications. A biopsy of the temporal artery should be obtained to confirm the clinical diagnosis of giant cell arteritis.

4. A healthy 48-year-old man complains of seeing "floating black dots" in the field of vision of his right eye for 2 days, associated with the sensation of brief flashing lights in the periphery of his visual field. He states that he has a disturbance in the temporal field of vision of his right eye, "like a curtain coming down." His visual acuity is OU 20/20. Pupils are normal. Confrontation visual field examination shows mild temporal visual field loss in the right eye only. Anterior segment exam is normal. The red reflex is clear in the left eye, but the red reflex in the right eye reveals opacities that are mobile. A retinal examination with the direct ophthalmoscope is normal. What is your course of action?

Answer: This patient needs prompt ophthalmologic consultation. The symptoms of new onset of floaters, flashing lights, and peripheral visual field loss are suggestive of retinal detachment. Floaters sometimes indicate red blood cells in the vitreous due to a retinal tear. Floaters may be visible to the patient but difficult to appreciate with the ophthalmoscope. If the vitreous blood is significant, it can be visualized in the red reflex as dark, mobile spots. Because the retina has no sensitivity to pain and is, in fact, limited to the sensation of light, the patient may report flashes of light as the retina tears or detaches. Retinal tears and early retinal detachments are usually located in the far periphery of the retina and may not be visible with the direct ophthalmoscope. In this patient, even though the initial examination is normal, the symptoms alone indicate the need for referral.

ANNOTATED RESOURCES

Beck RW, Cleary PA, Trobe JD, et al. The effect of corticosteroids for acute optic neuritis on the subsequent development of multiple sclerosis. The Optic Neuritis Study Group. *N Engl J Med.* 1993;329:1764–1769. In this multicenter randomized controlled clinical trial involving 389 patients without known multiple sclerosis, short-term, high-dose, intravenous corticosteroid administration appeared to reduce the rate of development of the disease over a 2-year period.

Miller NR, Newman NJ. *Walsh & Hoyt's Clinical Neuro-Ophthalmology.* 5th ed. Philadelphia, PA: Lippincott Williams & Wilkins; 1998. The second volume of this excellent 5-volume set provides an extensive discussion of disorders of the optic nerve.

Salvarani C, Cantini F, Boiardi L, et al. Polymyalgia rheumatica and giant cell arteritis. *N Engl J Med.* 2002;347:261–271. A review of ocular and systemic manifestation of these disorders.

Trobe JD. *The Physician's Guide to Eye Care.* 3rd ed. San Francisco, CA: American Academy of Ophthalmology; 2006. A concise yet comprehensive resource covering the principal clinical ophthalmic problems that nonophthalmologist physicians are likely to encounter, organized for practical use by practitioners.

Trobe JD. *The Neurology of Vision.* New York, NY: Oxford University Press; 2001. Part IV, chapters 10 through 15, presents retinal vascular, optic nerve, and cerebrovascular causes of acute visual loss.

Vaughan DG, Asbury T, Riordan-Eva P, eds. *General Ophthalmology.* 17th ed. Norwalk, CT: Appleton & Lange; 2007. The chapter on neuro-ophthalmology provides additional information on causes of acute visual loss.

Chronic Visual Loss

CHAPTER

3

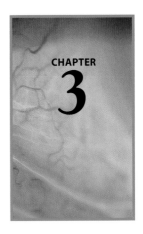

OBJECTIVES

As a primary care physician, you should be familiar with the major causes of chronic, slowly progressive visual loss in adult patients—namely, glaucoma, cataract, and macular degeneration—and be able to identify the basic characteristics of each. (See also Chapter 8 for a discussion of diabetic retinopathy, another important cause of chronic visual loss.) In addition, you should know the risk factors for glaucoma and be able to evaluate the optic nerve head, classifying it as normal, glaucomatous, or abnormal but nonglaucomatous. You also should be able to evaluate the clarity of the lens as well as the function and appearance of the macula. To achieve these objectives, you should learn to

- ➤ Recognize those characteristics of the optic disc useful in determining whether a given disc is normal or abnormal
- ➤ Recognize a cataract and determine its approximate potential effect on the patient's vision
- ➤ Determine whether a cataract is the only cause of a patient's visual decrease
- ➤ Examine the macula with the ophthalmoscope and recognize the signs and symptoms of maculopathy

CHRONIC VISUAL LOSS IN THE GERIATRIC POPULATION

In the United States, there are an estimated 4.7 million visually impaired persons and nearly 700,000 who are blind (WHO 2002 estimates). Age-related macular degeneration (AMD) leads cataract, glaucoma, and diabetes as the main causes of visual loss in the western population over age 50 (WHO 2002 data). By 2030, there will be 70 million Americans over age 65. Of these, 33% will develop a vision-altering disease. The elderly suffer disproportionately with increased prevalence and more severe loss of vision from eye disease. Approximately 82% of all people who are blind (about 37 million) are aged 50 and older, although they represent only 19% of the world's population (WHO 2002 estimates). Of those blind from glaucoma, 75% are over 65 years of age.

47

Visual loss has significant psychosocial, comorbid, and functional effects on the elderly. Twice as many community-dwelling adults with advanced AMD (20/60 or worse in the better eye) were diagnosed with major depression, compared to similar adults without visual loss. In Sweden, falls in those age 60 or older account for one-third of the total cost of medical care for all injuries. One study of falls in the Swedish residential population showed a fourfold increase in impaired vision in those who fell (28.8%) compared to those who did not (6.4%). Of "fallers" 32.7% sustained fracture, with 12% of falls resulting in fracture; more recurrent fallers (29.4%) had impaired vision, compared to "non-fallers" (14.3%). With aging there is increased risk of binocular functional acuity loss to less than 20/40, with a two-fold increase in blacks compared to whites. This decrease of acuity correlates with functional loss in activities of daily living and with social isolation after correction for age, gender, and race.

Age-related deficits in perceptual motor performance, motor ability, and reaction time compound the decreases in visual acuity, contrast sensitivity, and visual spatial attention. Consequently, the older driver is at increased risk of traffic accidents per mile. There is a loss in visuomotor tracking, eye movement excursions, and visual search with aging, although the elderly maintain their sustained attention with age. An elderly driver deemed at risk can be further evaluated by a "useful field of view" test, which assesses the person's ability to divide his or her attention from a central target to a briefly visible peripheral stimulus. A 40% impairment of the useful field of view test correlates with a 2.2-times increase in the likelihood of a motor vehicle accident. Impairment of the useful field of view has also been correlated with an increased risk of bodily injury to the driver and to others in a motor vehicle accident.

GLAUCOMA

Glaucoma is a significant cause of blindness in the United States and is the most frequent cause of blindness among African Americans. The incidence of glaucoma increases with advancing age and in patients with a family history of glaucoma. If glaucoma is detected early and treated medically or surgically, blindness can be prevented. Most patients with early glaucoma are asymptomatic. The great majority of patients lack pain, ocular inflammation, or halos (luminous or colored rings seen around lights). A significant amount of peripheral vision can be lost before the patient notices visual disability.

Glaucoma is usually insidious because symptoms and noticeable visual field defects occur in late stages of the disease process. Visual field defects are characterized by scotomas (areas of reduced or absent vision; see Figure 3.1) of various shape and a contraction of the peripheral field that usually spares the central vision until late in the disease process. Detection of glaucoma in the early asymptomatic stage requires an active effort, and it is very important because blindness can usually be prevented if treatment is adequate and timely.

Glaucoma often involves elevation of intraocular pressure (IOP) above the statistical range of 10 to 21 mm Hg in a non-gaussian distribution. Prolonged

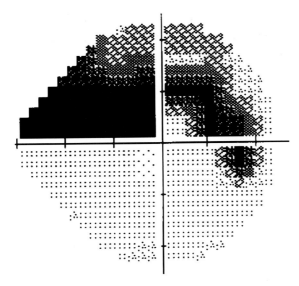

FIGURE 3.1 Superior arcuate scotoma as shown by automated visual field testing. (Courtesy Carla J. Siegfried, MD)

elevation of IOP can lead to optic nerve damage; however, in many cases, glaucomatous optic nerve changes are evident despite an apparently "normal" pressure (Figure 3.2). Therefore, examination of the optic nerve is the most important way to detect glaucoma in a primary care setting. Other disorders, such as an intracranial tumor, can also lead to changes in the optic nerve appearance; thus, the ability to recognize abnormalities of the optic nerve is an important skill for the primary care physician.

Measurement of IOP, an independent risk factor for glaucoma, is not a valuable means of screening for glaucoma. Glaucoma screenings that include formal (ie, automated, not manual confrontational) visual field analysis and examination of the optic nerve may be beneficial but are costly and require trained personnel. Thus, evaluation of risk factors (see Table 3.1) and examination of the optic nerve by the primary care physician with appropriate referral to the ophthalmologist are the best defenses against this silent, potentially blinding disease.

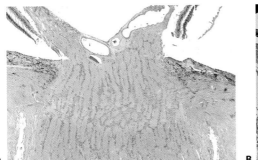
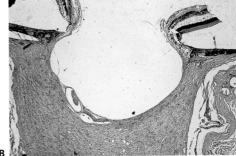

FIGURE 3.2 Pathologic sections, optic nerve. **A.** Longitudinal cross-section of normal optic nerve. (Courtesy University of Iowa, FC Blodi Eye Pathology Laboratory) **B.** Longitudinal cross-section of glaucomatous optic nerve showing enlarged cup and bean-pot excavation. (Courtesy Morton Smith, MD)

TABLE 3.1 Glaucoma Risk Factor Analysis: History-Based Risk Factor Weights

VARIABLE[a]	CATEGORY	WEIGHT
Age	< 50 years	0
	50–64 years	1
	65–74 years	2
	75 years	3
Race	Caucasian/other	0
	African American	2
Family history of glaucoma	Negative or positive in non–first-degree relatives	0
	Positive for parents	1
	Positive for siblings	2
Last complete eye examination	Within past 2 years	0
	2–5 years ago	1
	> 5 years ago	2

[a] Other historical variables, such as high myopia or hyperopia, systemic hypertension, corticosteroid use, and perhaps diabetes, are not strong enough to be assigned a weight but may be considered in the overall assessment of glaucoma risk.

LEVEL OF GLAUCOMA RISK	WEIGHTING SCORE
High	4 or greater (referral advisable)
Moderate	3 (referral advisable)
Low	2 or less

BASIC INFORMATION

This section reviews IOP, the types of glaucoma, the optic nerve, and the relationship of IOP to the optic nerve.

Intraocular Pressure

Within the eye is a mechanism for the continuous production and drainage of fluid. This fluid, called *aqueous humor*, is produced by the ciliary body of the eye. Aqueous humor flows through the pupil into the anterior chamber, where it is drained through the trabecular meshwork to Schlemm's canal (Figure 3.3), and onward to the venous system. Because of some resistance to the flow of aqueous through the trabecular meshwork and Schlemm's canal, pressure is created in the eye. All eyes have an internal pressure.

Intraocular pressure is largely dependent on the ease of flow through the trabecular meshwork and Schlemm's canal. The greater the resistance to flow, the higher the IOP. Although the eye contains several compartments, for purposes of pressure

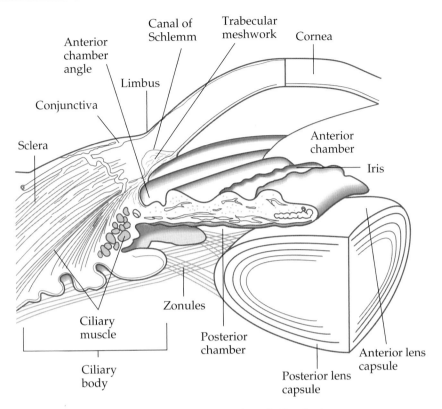

FIGURE 3.3 Cross-section of anterior chamber angle and ciliary body.

it can be considered a single closed space. Thus, the pressure exerted within the eye is equal over the entire wall of the eye. Most normal eyes have an IOP of 10–21 mm Hg (mean ±2 standard deviations).

Types of Glaucoma

In the common, insidious form of glaucoma, the chamber angle remains open. Accordingly, this form of glaucoma is called *open-angle glaucoma*. In rare instances, the trabecular meshwork can become suddenly and completely occluded by iris tissue. This causes an abrupt rise in IOP known *as acute angle-closure glaucoma* (see Figure 4.1) and constitutes an ocular emergency. The abrupt rise in pressure causes symptoms of pain, nausea, and colored halos or rainbows around light. *These symptoms do not occur in open-angle glaucoma.* An acute attack of angle closure usually produces a red, teary eye with a hazy cornea and a fixed, mid-dilated pupil. The eye feels extremely firm to palpation in most cases.

As opposed to acute angle-closure glaucoma, chronic angle-closure glaucoma has intermittent, low-grade symptoms of headache and blurred vision, especially in situations that induce pupillary dilation. Gradual scarring of the drainage angle occurs, resulting in elevated IOP.

Several developmental disorders can lead to elevated IOP that can result in early-onset glaucoma. Congenital or infantile glaucoma presents with tearing and sensitivity to light secondary to the corneal edema that results from highly elevated IOP. If the pressure remains elevated, the immature eye tissues expand and the eye enlarges (buphthalmos). In contrast, juvenile glaucoma presents a little later in life and is much more insidious, like the adult forms of the disease.

Glaucoma may be associated with other ocular disorders, systemic disease, medications, ocular trauma, and inflammation, and may occur following intraocular surgery. In addition, some forms of glaucoma have an identifiable genetic basis, but this currently accounts for a very small percentage of all patients with glaucoma.

Optic Nerve

The optic nerve is composed of more than 1.2 million nerve fibers. These nerve fibers originate in the ganglion cells of the retina, gather in a bundle as the optic nerve, and carry visual information to the brain. An interruption of these nerve fibers results in damage to vision.

The optic nerve can be seen at its origin by using the ophthalmoscope. At the point of origin, the nerve is called the *optic disc*. The optic disc often has a small depression in it called the *optic cup*. The size of the cup in normal eyes can vary with the individual. A complete description of the optic disc appears in Chapter 1.

Relationship of IOP and the Optic Nerve

Intraocular pressure is exerted on all "walls" of the eye, including the optic nerve and its blood vessels. The optic nerve is supplied with blood via branches of the ophthalmic artery, itself a branch of the internal carotid artery. Vascular disease may predispose patients to optic nerve damage. Thus, IOP-dependent and eye pressure-independent factors (eg, vascular disease) play a role in the development of glaucoma. Glaucoma is the general term used to describe the progressive optic neuropathy that can lead to blindness if untreated.

Glaucomatous optic neuropathy causes visual field loss. Early nerve damage usually causes localized peripheral visual field loss that is undetectable by the patient, but which can progress to impair central vision and eventually total vision if the disease is not adequately treated. Currently, all treatment regimens are directed toward lowering IOP. Measurement of IOP, evaluation of the optic nerve appearance, and visual field testing play a key role in diagnosis and monitoring of glaucoma.

WHEN TO EXAMINE

Ophthalmoscopy should be part of every comprehensive eye examination. Particular attention should be given to patients who are predisposed to glaucoma, such as elderly individuals or those with a family history of glaucoma. The American Academy of Ophthalmology recommends a glaucoma screening every 2 to 4 years past age 40, as the incidence of the disease increases with age. Because African Americans have an even greater risk for development of glaucoma, those between ages 20 and 39 should also be screened every 3 to 5 years.

HOW TO EXAMINE

Palpation can detect only very hard and very soft eyes; it is totally unreliable in the range of the most common glaucomatous intraocular pressures. Intraocular pressure is best measured via tonometry, which may be performed in any of several ways. Goldmann applanation tonometry is performed with a device connected to the slit lamp and is considered the "gold standard" for measurement. Hand-held tonometers (Tono-Pen) are available as are indentation, or Schiøtz, tonometers. Detailed information on various methods of tonometry appears in Chapter 1. The technique of direct ophthalmoscopy, also described in Chapter 1, is particularly useful in assessing the state of the optic disc.

An ophthalmologist evaluating a patient with suspected glaucoma will examine the anterior chamber angle structures using a special contact lens on the topically anesthetized cornea, a technique called *gonioscopy*. In addition, measurement of the central corneal thickness is important. Thin corneas result in artificially low IOP measurement, and thick corneas measure higher than the actual IOP. Corneal thickness has been shown to be an independent risk factor for the development of glaucoma. The ophthalmologist will also perform perimetry (automated visual field testing). Finally, documentation of the optic nerve appearance for future comparison is performed with stereo disc photography or other forms of optic nerve analysis.

HOW TO INTERPRET THE FINDINGS

The appearance of the optic disc can be described generally in terms of its color and of the size of its physiologic cup (a recognizable central depression within the optic disc). The color of the optic nerve can be important in determining atrophy of the nerve that is due to glaucoma or other causes. Temporal pallor of the optic nerve (Figure 3.4) can occur as a result of diseases that damage the nerve fibers, such as brain tumors or optic nerve inflammation, or in conjunction with glaucomatous cupping.

The term *glaucomatous cupping* refers to an increase in the size of the optic cup relative to the optic disc that occurs in glaucoma. The increase in the cup is due to loss of nerve fibers bundled in the optic nerve. The so-called *cup:disc ratio* is determined by comparing the diameter of the cup to that of the disc (Figure 3.5). The optic discs generally should appear symmetric between the eyes, and asymmetric cup:disc ratios should arouse suspicion of glaucoma. The larger the cup, the greater the probability of a glaucomatous optic nerve. A cup measuring one half the size of the disc or larger—a cup:disc ratio of 0.5 or more—raises suspicion of glaucoma (Figure 3.6). Disc hemorrhages (Figure 3.7) are also a possible sign of glaucoma. A large cup should be suspected if central pallor of the disc is prominent. Because the cup is a depressed area of the disc, retinal vessels passing over the disc are seen to bend at the edge of the cup, a useful sign in evaluating cup size. Vessel displacement, then, as well as disc color, should be evaluated in determining the size of the cup (Figure 3.8).

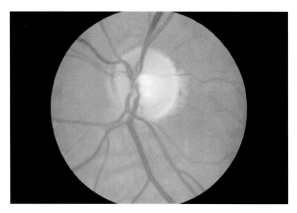

FIGURE 3.4 Temporal pallor of the optic nerve. Diseases that damage optic nerve fibers may result in temporal pallor of the optic nerve. Note the normal nerve color present only on the nasal aspect of the disc.

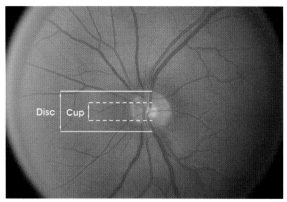

FIGURE 3.5 Cup:disc ratio. In this nondiseased optic disc, the cup is less than one-half the diameter of the disc, indicating absent or low level of suspicion of glaucoma.

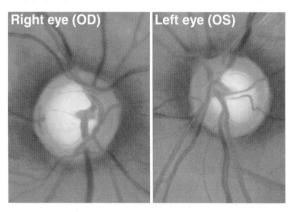

FIGURE 3.6 Glaucomatous cupping. Patient's right eye shows a cup:disc ratio of 0.8 (high level of glaucoma suspicion); the left eye shows a cup:disc ratio of 0.6 (moderate level of glaucoma suspicion). The asymmetry of cup:disc ratios here also raises suspicion of glaucoma.

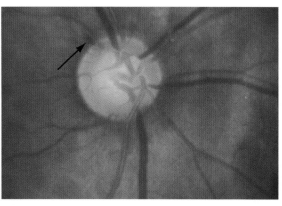

FIGURE 3.7 Disc hemorrhage. A hemorrhage on the optic disc may indicate glaucomatous damage.

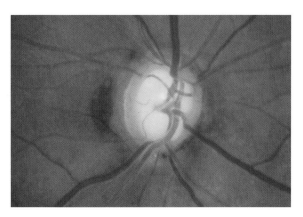

FIGURE 3.8 Glaucomatous optic atrophy. Optic nerve cupping is increased vertically, with a cup:disc ratio of 0.8. Cupping is apparent at the point where the vessels disappear over the edge of the attenuated rim.

MANAGEMENT OR REFERRAL

Table 3.1 provides a convenient method of analyzing a patient's level of glaucoma risk. A moderate or high level of glaucoma risk warrants referral to an ophthalmologist for further evaluation. In addition, any patient who has 1 or more of the following conditions should be referred to an ophthalmologist:

- Symptoms of acute glaucoma (Refer immediately; also see Figure 4.1.)
- An optic cup diameter one half or more of the disc diameter (ie, a cup:disc ratio of 0.5 or greater)
- Cup:disc asymmetry of more than 0.1 between the 2 optic nerves (eg, right eye 0.4, left eye 0.2)

For a discussion of systemic side effects of topically administered drugs used in the treatment of glaucoma, see Chapter 9.

CATARACT

Cataract may occur as a congenital or genetic anomaly, as a result of various diseases, or with increasing age. Some degree of cataract formation is to be expected in all people over age 70. In fact, age-related cataract occurs in about 50% of people between ages 65 and 74 and in about 70% of those over 75.

Cataract is the most common cause of decreased vision (not correctable with glasses) in the United States. However, it is one of the most successfully treated conditions in all of surgery. Approximately 1.64 million cataract extractions are done each year in the United States, usually with implantation of an intraocular lens. If an implant is not used, visual rehabilitation is still possible with a contact lens or thick (aphakic) eyeglasses.

If cataract surgery is considered, it is important to be certain that visual loss is explained fully by cataract or significantly by the cataract if other ocular conditions such as glaucoma, macular degeneration, or diabetic retinopathy are also present. Assessment of the visual significance of the cataract is more difficult with coexisting ocular pathology. Sometimes cataract surgery is performed to facilitate diagnosis or treatment of other ocular diseases.

BASIC INFORMATION

This section provides an overview of the lens as well as cataracts and their symptoms.

Lens

The crystalline lens focuses a clear image on the retina. The lens is suspended by thin filamentous zonules from the ciliary body between the iris anteriorly and the vitreous humor posteriorly. Contraction of the ciliary muscle permits focusing of the lens. The lens is enclosed in a capsule of transparent elastic basement membrane. The capsule encloses the cortex and the nucleus of the lens as well as a single anterior layer of cuboidal epithelium. The lens has no innervation or blood supply. Nourishment comes from the aqueous fluid and the vitreous.

The normal lens continues to grow throughout life. The epithelial cells continue to produce new cortical lens fibers, yielding a slow increase in size, weight, and density over the years. The normal lens consists of 35% protein by mass. The percentage of insoluble protein increases as the lens ages and as a cataract develops.

Cataracts

A cataract is any opacity or discoloration of the lens, whether a small, local opacity or the complete loss of transparency. Clinically, the term *cataract* is usually reserved for opacities that affect visual acuity because many normal lenses have small, visually insignificant opacities.

A cataract is described in terms of the zones of the lens involved in the opacity. These zones of opacity may be subcapsular, cortical, or nuclear and may be anterior or posterior in location. In addition to opacification of the nucleus and cortex, there may be a yellow or amber color change to the lens. A cataract also can be described in terms of its stage of development. A cataract with a clear cortex remaining is immature. A mature cataract (Figure 3.9) has a totally opacified cortex.

The most common cause of cataract is age-related change. Other causative factors include trauma, inflammation, metabolic and nutritional defects, and the effects of corticosteroids. Cataracts may develop very slowly over years or may progress rapidly, depending on the cause and type of cataract.

Symptoms of Cataract

Patients may first notice image blur as the lens loses its ability to resolve separate and distinct objects. Patients are first aware of a disturbance of vision, then a diminution, and finally a failure of vision. The degree of visual disability caused by a cataract depends on the size and location of the opacity. Axial opacities—affecting the nucleus or central subcapsular areas—cause much more disabling visual loss than do peripheral opacities.

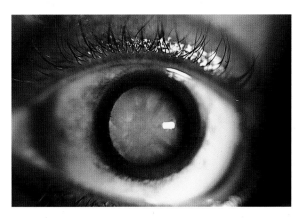

FIGURE 3.9 Mature cataract. A cataract is called mature when the lens is totally opacified. A red reflex cannot be obtained; the pupil appears white. The radial spokes in this figure reflect variations in density of the radially arranged fibers in the cortical layers of the lens. Light still reaching the retina is totally diffused and will allow the perception of light but not form.

Patients with nuclear sclerosis may develop increasing lenticular (ie, referring to the crystalline lens) myopia because of the increased refractive power of the denser nucleus. As the size of the cataract increases, patients become progressively more myopic. Patients may find they can read without the glasses normally required, a phenomenon often called *second sight*. Patients may note monocular double or multiple images, due to irregular refraction within the lens. They frequently complain of "starbursts" around lights and difficulty with night driving. With yellowing of the lens nucleus, objects appear browner or yellower and color discrimination is more difficult.

Patients with posterior subcapsular cataracts (Figure 3.10) may note a relatively rapid decrease in vision, with glare as well as image blur and distortion. In contrast to nuclear cataracts (Figure 3.11), posterior subcapsular cataracts frequently affect near vision. This type of cataract may be associated with metabolic causes such as diabetes mellitus or corticosteroid use.

Over time, cataracts may lead to a generalized impairment of vision. The degree of visual disability often varies depending on lighting and tasks the patient needs to perform.

WHEN TO EXAMINE

A patient with decreasing vision requires a complete examination to determine the cause of the visual decline. Evaluation of the visual significance of a cataract includes optic nerve and retinal evaluation to detect coexisting disease that could also affect the visual acuity. Special attention is given to the macula when a patient reports difficulty with near work or metamorphopsia (ie, a wavy distortion of central vision). In the presence of coexisting disease, the ophthalmologist may order special tests to better determine the contribution of the cataract to the decreased visual acuity.

If the lens is densely cataractous, the ophthalmoscope will not provide a view of the fundus through the opacity. In this situation, retinal and optic nerve pathology cannot be adequately assessed. For example, if the patient has diabetic retinopathy in the contralateral eye, there is increased risk for a portion of the visual loss in the

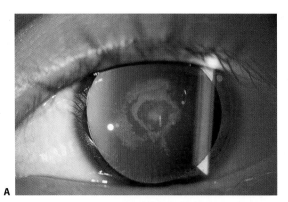

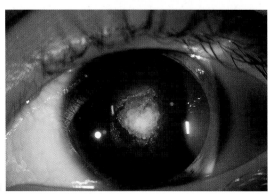

FIGURE 3.10 Posterior subcapsular cataract. **A.** The red reflex has a central dark shadow. **B.** Posterior subcapsular cataracts can be seen in younger patients and may be associated with chronic steroid use. (Courtesy Cynthia A. Bradford, MD)

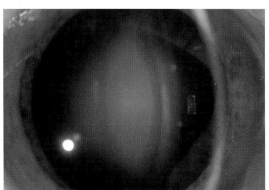

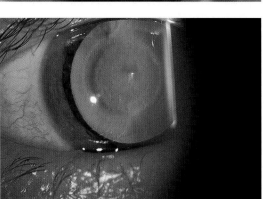

FIGURE 3.11 Nuclear cataract. **A.** Slit-lamp photograph of nuclear sclerotic cataract demonstrates the yellow coloration of the cataract and the central granular opacification. **B.** Red reflex photograph of the same cataract highlights the central distortion of the lens that results in the decreased visual acuity as well as the phenomenon of starbursts around lights. This can easily be seen with the direct ophthalmoscope if the pupil is dilated. (Courtesy Cynthia A. Bradford, MD)

eye with cataract to be related to diabetic retinopathy. Removal of the cataract would allow evaluation and possible treatment of the retinal pathology. The patient should understand the expected visual outcome of surgery.

HOW TO EXAMINE

The following examination methods are helpful in obtaining an accurate history of visual decline and determining whether visual loss is attributable to cataract, to some other cause, or to a combination of causes.

Visual Acuity Testing

The first step in any evaluation of visual decrease is the measurement of visual acuity. Refer to Chapter 1 for details.

Pupillary Reaction Testing

Chapter 7 describes how to perform a basic pupillary examination and provides details on the neurologic implications of pupillary responses. Even an advanced cataract would not produce a relative afferent pupillary defect.

Slit-Lamp Examination

The examination at the slit lamp provides a magnified view of the lens, aiding in the description of the type, severity, and location of the cataract. Assessment of the red reflex can also assist with identification of posterior subcapsular cataracts and other axial opacities. The integrity of the zonular support of the lens can also be determined by slit-lamp exam.

Ophthalmoscopy

Although it is difficult to accurately predict the effect of the cataract on the patient's visual acuity and function, the view of the fundus is usually obscured to some extent by very dense opacities, especially with the direct ophthalmoscope and slit-lamp biomicroscopy. Funduscopic examination is required to evaluate the macula and optic nerve for disease that could be contributing to the visual loss. If the cataract completely obscures the fundus view, ultrasonography may be required to evaluate the posterior segment of the eye.

HOW TO INTERPRET THE FINDINGS

An early cataract is not visible to the unaided eye. If the cataract becomes very dense, it may appear as a white pupil, or leukocoria. The lens can be evaluated with the ophthalmoscope using a plus-lens setting. The lens opacification with a partial cataract will appear black against the red reflex of the fundus. Generally, the denser the cataract, the poorer the red reflex and the worse the visual acuity. It is important not to assign visual loss to cataract before ensuring that other, more serious causes of visual loss have not been overlooked.

MANAGEMENT OR REFERRAL

The decision to refer a patient with cataract should be based in part on whether or not the cataract keeps the patient from doing what he or she wants to do. A cataract can interfere with patients' activities of daily living by limiting their ability to drive safely, read, or participate in sports or other hobbies. Patients with cataract-associated visual loss that negatively affects their daily living may benefit from a surgical procedure of cataract extraction with intraocular lens implantation. A prospective study has shown that cataract extraction is associated with a 50% drop in motor vehicle accidents. Uncorrected, chronic visual loss in older patients in residential care has been associated with an increased risk of falls and falling injuries. The Framingham Study found an increase in the relative risk of hip fracture with moderate (20/30 to 20/80) and severe (20/100 or worse) vision impairment over 10 years of 1.54 and 2.17, respectively. Even moderate vision loss in one eye alone was associated with an increased risk of 1.94, suggesting the role of good stereoscopic vision in prevention of falls and fractures.

After cataract extraction surgery, many patients require a laser surgical procedure to open an opacified posterior capsule. This has led to a popular misconception that a cataract can actually be removed with a laser. The operating surgeon should preoperatively examine all patients who are contemplating cataract surgery. A discussion with the surgeon on the risks and benefits of, and the alternatives to, the surgery, as well as planning for postoperative care, is imperative.

MACULAR DEGENERATION

In the United States, age-related macular degeneration (AMD) is the leading cause of irreversible central visual loss (20/200 or worse) among people age 50 or older. Because certain types of macular degeneration can be effectively treated, it is important to recognize this entity and to refer for appropriate care. It is important to distinguish between the possible causes of visual loss, whether cataract (surgically correctable), glaucoma (medically or surgically treatable), or macular degeneration (potentially treatable medically or by laser surgery).

BASIC INFORMATION

This section introduces macular anatomy and macular changes due to aging.

Macular Anatomy

The macula is situated between the temporal vascular arcades. The center of the macula, the fovea, is an oval area situated about 2 disc diameters temporal and slightly inferior to the optic disc (see Figure 1.15 for a depiction of the normal fundus). The macula is composed of both rods and cones and is the area responsible for detailed, fine central vision. The fovea (Figure 3.12) is partly avascular and appears darker than the surrounding retina. The foveola is the pit-like depression in the center of the macula. Here, there is a high density of cones but no rods are

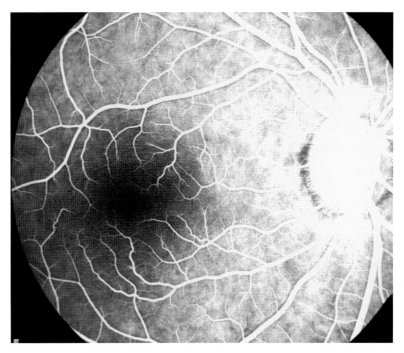

FIGURE 3.12   Fovea. The fovea is avascular, as demonstrated in this fundus fluorescein angiogram. The central capillary-free zone identifies the foveal region. (Courtesy Reagan Bradford, MD)

present. The central depression of the fovea may act like a concave mirror during ophthalmoscopy, producing a light reflection (ie, foveal reflex).

Age-Related Macular Changes

Macular changes due to age include drusen, degenerative changes in the retinal pigment epithelium, and choroidal neovascular membranes.

Drusen are hyaline nodules (or colloid bodies) deposited in Bruch's membrane, which separates the retinal pigment epithelium (the outermost layer of the retina) from the inner choroidal vessels. Drusen may be small and discrete (Figure 3.13) or larger, with irregular shapes and indistinct edges. Patients with drusen alone tend to have normal or near-normal visual acuity, with minimal metamorphopsia. Drusen may be seen with increasing age, with retinal or choroidal degeneration, and as a primary dystrophy.

Degenerative changes in the retinal pigment epithelium itself may occur with or without drusen. These degenerative changes are manifested as clumps of hyperpigmentation or depigmented atrophic areas (Figure 3.14). The effect on visual acuity is variable.

About 20% of eyes with age-related macular degeneration develop choroidal neovascularization, producing the so-called *neovascular*, or "wet," macular degeneration. The extension of vessels from the inner choroid layer into the sub-pigment

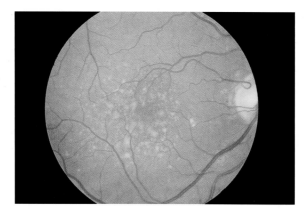

FIGURE 3.13 Drusen. Small and medium-sized drusen (yellow deposits) are visible beneath the right macula in this patient with nonexudative, or "dry," age-related macular degeneration. Although acuity may be normal initially, these lesions can lead to significant visual loss if the central macula becomes involved. (Courtesy Ronald M. Kingsley, MD)

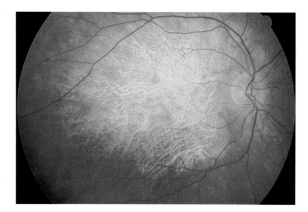

FIGURE 3.14 Retinal pigment epithelial atrophy. An extensive area of geographic, submacular pigment atrophy involves the entire posterior retina between the temporal retinal vascular arcades. The underlying choroidal vasculature is more prominent when the pigment epithelium is absent or atrophic. This patient demonstrates advanced nonexudative age-related macular degeneration. Such a patient typically has poor visual acuity. (Courtesy Ronald M. Kingsley, MD)

epithelial space and eventually into the subretinal space occurs through a defect in Bruch's membrane.

The choroidal neovascular net may be associated with subretinal hemorrhage and exudates (Figure 3.15), and with fibrosis in the late or disciform stage. Subretinal hemorrhage may result in acute visual loss (see Chapter 2). The larger the membrane and the closer to the center of the fovea, the worse the prognosis for good central vision.

Fluorescein angiography, a technique utilized by ophthalmologists, may be necessary to identify neovascularization and is mandatory before considering laser surgery. Intravenous injection of fluorescein dye and subsequent rapid-sequence photography help demonstrate the retinal and choroidal vasculature. In contrast

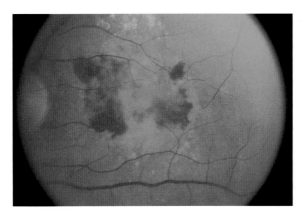

FIGURE 3.15 Subretinal hemorrhage. The subfoveal fluid, hemorrhage, and exudate present in this patient indicate choroidal neovascularization. These findings are often present in patients with neovascular, or "wet," age-related macular degeneration. (Courtesy Ronald M. Kingsley, MD)

to competent retinal veins and arteries, new vessels can be identified because they leak fluorescein dye. In addition, because the retinal pigment epithelium normally acts as a physical and optical barrier to fluorescein, angiography facilitates identification of pigment epithelial defects. Indocyanine green is another dye used to demonstrate choroidal neovascularization.

Ocular coherence tomography (OCT), a newer imaging technology, is a noninvasive method to image retinal structures in vivo. Cross-sectional images are produced that display the anatomic layers of the retina and measurements of retinal thickness.

Compare Figure 3.15, a fundus photograph depicting a subretinal hemorrhage implying the presence of choroidal neovascularization, with Figure 3.16, a fundus fluorescein angiogram of the same eye, which reveals the choroidal neovascularization and associated subretinal hemorrhage. Figure 3.17 is an OCT image of choroidal neovascularization and subretinal fluid.

Age-related changes are typically confined to the posterior pole of the eye. Thus, the patient with AMD may have very poor central vision but tends to retain functional peripheral vision. Visual aids, such as high-plus magnifiers and telescopic devices, may help the patient. In addition to age, other causes of chronic maculopathy include heredity and metabolic changes.

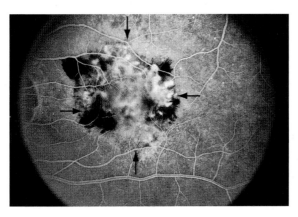

FIGURE 3.16 Neovascular net. The fluorescein frame depicts the neovascular net in the fundus photograph in Figure 3.15. The hyperfluorescent (bright) area under the left fovea highlights the area of neovascularization and is used to determine the management strategy. (Courtesy Ronald M. Kingsley, MD)

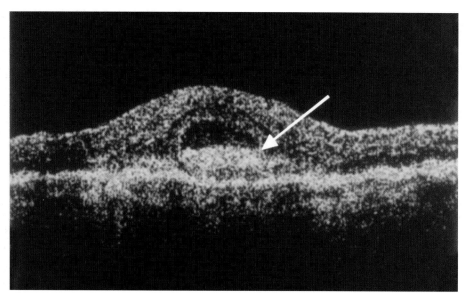

FIGURE 3.17 Optical coherence tomography (OCT) imaging shows the choroidal neovascularization as a discrete reflective, subretinal lesion (white arrow) above the retinal pigment epithelium. Subretinal and intraretinal fluid is also present. (Reprinted with permission from Elsevier. Hughes EH et al. In vivo demonstration of the anatomic differences between classic and occult choroidal neovascularization using optical coherence tomography. *Am J Ophthalmol.* 2005;139:345.)

WHEN TO EXAMINE

Any patient with decreasing vision requires examination to determine the cause of the visual change. In assessing a patient with blurred or distorted central vision, every effort should be made to examine the macula with the ophthalmoscope. Of course, opacities in the cornea, lens, or vitreous may preclude an adequate view of the macula.

HOW TO EXAMINE

The following techniques are especially helpful in evaluating macular degeneration as the cause of visual decrease or major changes in central vision.

Visual Acuity Measurement

Refer to Chapter 1 for instructions.

Amsler Grid Testing

Amsler grid testing (Figure 3.18) is a useful method of evaluating the function of the macula. Utilizing a patient's best near correction, the test is carried out by having the patient look with one eye at a time at a central spot on a page where horizontal and vertical parallel lines make up a square grid pattern. This grid pattern may be printed with white lines against a black background or vice versa. The patient is asked to note irregularities in the lines. Irregularities may be reported as lines that are wavy, seem to bow or bend, appear gray or fuzzy, or are absent in

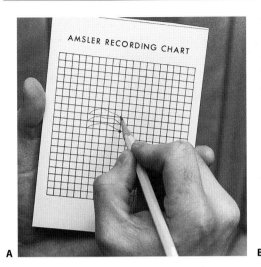
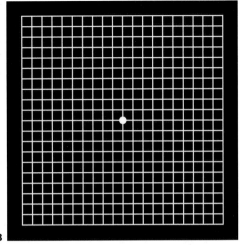

FIGURE 3.18 Amsler grid testing. **A.** The patient indicates the nature and location of his central field defect by sketching what he perceives on the Amsler grid. **B.** The typical grid pattern of white lines on a black background.

certain areas of the grid, indicating a scotoma. The straight line, right angle, and square are geometric shapes that highlight areas of distortions most easily. With the chart held at a normal reading distance of 30 cm from the eye, the Amsler grid tests the central 20° of visual field. Thus, the entire macula is evaluated with this examination.

Ophthalmoscopy

The macular area is studied with the direct ophthalmoscope. Sometimes it is helpful to have the patient look directly into the light of the instrument. Dilation of the pupil is usually necessary for adequate examination.

Additional Studies

The ophthalmologist may elect to carry out special studies to better evaluate the macula and macular function. Procedures such as stereoscopic slit-lamp examination, fluorescein angiography, and OCT may be necessary to determine pathologic changes.

HOW TO INTERPRET THE FINDINGS

The appearance of the macula often does not accurately predict the visual acuity. The macula may look more or less involved than the vision indicates. Drusen, areas of decreased or increased pigmentation, subretinal exudate, and hemorrhage are all important signs to check for in a direct ophthalmoscopic examination of the macula. The absence of the foveal reflex and a mottled appearance of the underlying retinal pigment epithelium are among the early signs of macular disease.

MANAGEMENT OR REFERRAL

Any patient who has 1 or more of the following should be referred to an ophthalmologist:

- Recent onset of decreased visual acuity
- Recent onset of metamorphopsia (central visual distortion)
- Recent onset of a scotoma (blind spot)
- Any ophthalmoscopic abnormalities in the appearance of the macula, such as drusen, degenerative changes in the retinal pigment epithelium, exudate, or blood

Although a patient with metamorphopsia may have only drusen in the macula, many patients with this complaint have complicating choroidal neovascularization and most need fluorescein angiography and/or OCT to establish their diagnosis and management. Early clinical studies indicated that argon laser photocoagulation of choroidal neovascular membranes that are not too close to the fovea significantly reduces the risk of central visual loss. Treatments for neovascular AMD have dramatically improved since the Macular Photocoagulation Study in 1999. Permanent loss of central vision was often a result of the treatment to limit the spread of neovascularization. The availability of photodynamic therapy (PDT) with verteporfin (Visudyne) in 2000 allowed for selective photochemical damage to choroidal neovascularization with less collateral retinal and choroidal damage. However, 30% to 40% of patients still lost significant central vision.

The advent of newer anti–vascular endothelial growth factor (anti-VEGF) agents has resulted in improved visual outcomes. Specifically, ranibizumab (Lucentis) and bevacizumab (off-label use of Avastin) have been shown to reduce retinal thickness and improve visual acuity.

Because many of the available treatments are costly, the patient with neovascular AMD needs to carefully assess the existing evidence for treatment effectiveness before proceeding. Current therapies for neovascular AMD offer hope for patients with acute symptoms of visual loss (usually less than 3 months' duration). After several months, it is unlikely that treatment will benefit the patient visually.

There is ongoing research on the effect of vitamins on the development and progression of AMD. Although not yet a proven therapy, patients at risk for the development of AMD may be encouraged to eat a diet rich in green (kale, collard greens, spinach, broccoli) and yellow (corn, squash) vegetables as well as to take a daily multivitamin. They should also be cautioned that smoking is associated with more severe AMD.

Although there is currently no scientific evidence to support the use of antioxidant vitamins or mineral supplements to prevent the onset of AMD, the Age-Related Eye Disease Study (AREDS) provides evidence that these supplements reduce the progression of the dry and slowly progressing form of AMD to the wet form with acute vision loss. Consequently, patients who are 50 years of age or older with high-risk drusen should be evaluated by an ophthalmologist to consider their need for oral supplementation with a daily dose of antioxidants (500 mg of vitamin C, 400 IU of vitamin E, and 15 mg of beta carotene) and minerals (80 mg of zinc oxide and 2 mg of cupric oxide) to reduce the risk of progressive vision loss from neovascular macular degeneration or geographic atrophy. This regimen is modified for smokers to exclude beta carotene because it may increase their risk of developing lung cancer.

THE VISUALLY IMPAIRED PATIENT

Despite medical or surgical therapy, some patients will have a significant residual visual impairment. These patients are candidates for low vision services and should be referred to an ophthalmologist capable of supplying these services. More than 11 million Americans have visual impairment that interferes with routine activities; 1.5 million are classified as severely visually handicapped. The use of visual aids will allow many of these patients to continue to function independently. The appropriate and timely intervention by the low vision specialist is an important part of patients' rehabilitation and should be considered a continuation of their ongoing medical therapy.

POINTS TO REMEMBER

- Glaucoma should be suspected when ophthalmoscopy reveals either prominent cupping of the optic discs or significant asymmetry of the cup:disc ratio.
- The primary indication for cataract extraction in most patients is interference with the daily pattern of living rather than reduction of visual acuity to a particular level.
- Both treatment of neovascular membranes and low vision aids can be helpful to patients with AMD.

SAMPLE PROBLEMS

1. A 72-year-old African American woman with hypertension and type 2 diabetes mellitus comes to your office for a scheduled annual complete physical exam. Your review of systems reveals that her last complete eye exam was more than 10 years ago. She states that she has never worn glasses and is happy with over-the-counter reading glasses for reading fine print. She states that everyone in her family has "healthy" eyes and no one wears glasses. What is your recommendation?

   a. Continue present management. If her vision is fine, over-the-counter reading glasses are acceptable.

   b. Review symptoms of vision changes associated with diabetes, cataract, and glaucoma; if the patient denies any problems, continue present management.

c. Refer the patient to an ophthalmologist.

d. Check vision, do a fundus exam in the office, and, if negative, continue present management.

Answer: c. This patient should have a comprehensive ophthalmic examination at least annually for 2 reasons. As a diabetic, she should have a dilated fundus exam annually to screen for diabetic retinopathy. She also has 3 history-based risk factors for glaucoma: age, race, and last complete exam more than 5 years ago.

2. A retired patient of yours is developing a nuclear sclerotic cataract, and his visual acuity has decreased to OD 20/30 and OS 20/40. His vision bothers him while he is driving because he cannot read street signs. He went to an optometrist for new glasses but was told he needed cataract surgery. He was referred for cataract surgery in 1 week with a surgeon who has not examined his eyes. The optometrist suggested that he (the optometrist) perform the postoperative care, an arrangement called "comanagement." The patient asks your advice. What do you tell him?

a. Proceed with the surgery to help prevent a car accident.

b. Advise him to ask the surgeon to perform the postoperative care.

c. Advise him to seek a second opinion from an ophthalmologist who performs cataract surgery.

Answer: c. The decision to perform cataract surgery includes preoperative evaluation of all aspects of the eye to determine the impact of the cataract on the decreased visual acuity. For each patient, the operating surgeon must discuss the risk factors as well as the potential benefits of the surgery. The patient can then decide if he or she is interested in pursuing this elective surgery. Meeting the surgeon immediately before surgery does not allow the patient to make an unpressured decision. When situations arise in which the surgeon, in consultation with the patient and comanaging practitioner, concludes that the delegation of postoperative care is in the patient's best interest, it is recommended that the surgeon follow these steps:

1. Document the patient's free choice of postoperative provider after informed consent.

2. Ensure that the transfer of care does not occur until it is clinically appropriate and in the patient's best interest.

3. Confirm that the comanager is legally entitled and professionally trained to provide the particular services.

4. Inform the patient of the financial implications resulting from the comanagement arrangement, particularly with regard to the patient's payment obligations and the postoperative provider's reimbursement.

5. Reassure the patient that he or she has access to the surgeon, if necessary, during the postoperative period at no additional cost. Situations in which

patients might consider postoperative care by someone other than the surgeon might include patient or surgeon illness, or inability to travel. The decision to comanage should be the result of a determination of what is best for the patient and not economic considerations.

3. A 76-year-old man has noted visual distortion over the past week. His concern increased when he discovered that the distortion was in the right eye only. Straight lines viewed through his left eye remained straight, but they appeared to dip down in the center when viewed with his right eye only. Visual acuity testing revealed OD 20/50, OS 20/20.

   A. What further tests will help determine the source of the patient's visual loss?

   Answer: Amsler grid testing will document the patient's symptoms of metamorphopsia. Dilated fundus examination may reveal macular drusen, retinal hemorrhages secondary to subretinal neovascular membranes, or retinal pigment epithelial atrophy as a manifestation of age-related macular degeneration.

   B. What techniques do ophthalmologists use to identify neovascularization in consideration for treatment?

   Answer: Fluorescein angiography and OCT are used to document neovascularization and subretinal fluid.

   C. What percentage of patients with AMD develop subretinal neovascularization?

   Answer: Twenty percent of patients with AMD develop subretinal neovascularization.

ANNOTATED RESOURCES

Age-Related Eye Disease Study Research Group. A randomized, placebo-controlled, clinical trial of high-dose supplementation with vitamins C and E, beta carotene, and zinc for age-related macular degeneration and vision loss. *Arch Ophthalmol.* 2001;119:1417–1436.

Allingham RR, Shields MB. *Textbook of Glaucoma.* 5th ed. Baltimore, MD: Lippincott Williams & Wilkins; 2005. An excellent reference covering current medical and surgical therapies of the primary and secondary glaucomas.

Bressler NM and the Treatment of Age-Related Macular Degeneration with Photodynamic Therapy (TAP) Study Group. Photodynamic therapy of subfoveal choroidal neovascularization in age-related macular degeneration with verteporfin: 2-year results of 2 randomized clinical trials—TAP report 2. *Arch Ophthalmol.* 2001;119:198–207.

Brody BL, Bamst AC, Williams RA, et al. Depression, visual acuity, comorbidity, and disability associated with age-related macular degeneration. *Ophthalmology*. 2001;108:1893–1902.

Felson DT, Anderson JJ, Hannan MT, et al. Impaired vision and hip fracture, The Framingham Study. *J Am Geriatr Soc*. 1989;37:495–500.

Harvey PT. Common eye diseases of elderly people: identifying and treating causes of vision loss. *Gerontology*. 2003;49:1–11.

Jaffe NS, Jaffe MS, Jaffe GF. *Cataract Surgery and Its Complications*. 6th ed. St Louis, MO: CV Mosby Co; 1997. An excellent text covering the contemporary methods of surgical management of cataracts, including phacoemulsification, and the major intraoperative and postoperative complications associated with this surgery.

Kallin K, Lundin-Olsson L, Jensen J, et al. Predisposing and precipitating factors for falls among older people in residential care. *Public Health*. 2002;116:263–271.

Kaiser PK, Brown DM, Zhang K, et al. Ranibizumab for predominantly classic neovascular age-related macular degeneration: subgroup analysis of first-year ANCHOR results. *Am J Ophthalmol*. 2007;144:850–857.

Macular Photocoagulation Study Group. Argon laser photocoagulation for neovascular maculopathy: 3-year results from randomized clinical trials. *Arch Ophthalmol*. 1986;104:694–701. The beneficial effects of argon laser photocoagulation are demonstrated in eyes with an extrafoveal choroidal neovascular membrane.

Mangione CM, Phillips RS, Lawrence MG, et al. Improved visual function and attenuation of declines in health-related quality of life after cataract extraction. *Arch Ophthalmol*. 1994;112:1419–1425. Improved visual function after cataract surgery was associated with better health-related quality of life, suggesting that age-related declines in health may be attenuated by improvements in visual function.

Owsley C, McGwin G Jr, Sloane ME, et al. Impact of cataract surgery on motor vehicle crash involvement by older adults. *JAMA*. 2002;288:841–849.

Quigley HA. Current and future approaches to glaucoma screening. *J Glaucoma*. 1998;7:210–220. A nice review of the challenges of glaucoma screening with cost, sensitivity, and specificity analysis of various devices and techniques.

Tasman W, Jaeger EA, eds. *Duane's Ophthalmology*. CD-ROM. 15th ed. Philadelphia, PA: Lippincott Williams & Wilkins; 2009. "Diseases of the Lens" in Volume 1 provides basic background material on the anatomy, embryology, and physiology of the lens as well as the pathogenesis of cataract. "Glaucoma" in Volume 3 provides information on contemporary concepts about the glaucomas and their treatment. Both basic and advanced information is available in this volume. Chapter 23 in Volume 3 covers acquired macular disease, providing current information on AMD.

Trobe JD. *The Physician's Guide to Eye Care*. 3rd ed. San Francisco: American Academy of Ophthalmology; 2006. A brief but comprehensive resource covering the principal clinical ophthalmic problems that nonophthalmologist physicians are likely to encounter, organized for practical use by practitioners.

Verteporfin In Photodynamic Therapy Study Group. Verteporfin therapy of subfoveal choroidal neovascularization in age-related macular degeneration: 2-year results of a randomized clinical trial including lesions with occult with no classic choroidal neovascularization—verteporfin in photodynamic therapy report 2. *Am J Ophthalmol*. 2001;131:541–560.

West SK, Munoz B, Rubin G, et al. Function and visual impairment in a population-based study of older adults. The SEE project. Salisbury Eye Evaluation. *Invest Ophthalmol Vis Sci*. 1997;38:72–82.

The Red Eye

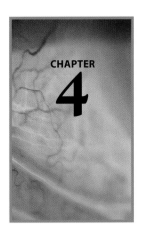

OBJECTIVES

As a primary care physician, you should be able to determine whether a patient with a red eye requires the prompt attention of an ophthalmologist or whether you can appropriately evaluate and treat the condition. To achieve this objective, you should learn to

➤ Obtain an accurate ocular history
➤ Perform the 9 basic diagnostic steps
➤ Recognize the danger signs of a red eye
➤ Describe the treatment for those cases you can manage and recognize the more serious problems that should be referred
➤ Describe the serious complications of prolonged use of topical anesthetic drops and of corticosteroids

RELEVANCE

A primary care physician frequently encounters patients who complain of a red eye. The condition causing the red eye is often a simple disorder such as a sub-conjunctival hemorrhage or an infectious conjunctivitis. These conditions either will resolve spontaneously or can be treated easily by the primary care physician. Occasionally, the condition causing a red eye is a more serious disorder, such as in-traocular inflammation, corneal inflammation, or acute glaucoma. A patient with one of these vision-threatening conditions requires the immediate attention of an ophthalmologist, whose specialized skills, knowledge, and examining instruments are needed in order to make correct therapeutic decisions.

BASIC INFORMATION

Red eye refers to *hyperemia,* or injection of the superficially visible vessels, of the conjunctiva, episclera, or sclera. Hyperemia can be caused by disorders of these structures or of adjoining structures, including the cornea, iris, ciliary body, and ocular adnexa. Specific disorders are discussed in the next section.

DISORDERS ASSOCIATED WITH A RED EYE

Any patient who complains of a red or painful eye should be examined to diagnose the condition as one of the following.

Acute Angle-Closure Glaucoma

Acute angle-closure glaucoma is an uncommon form of glaucoma due to sudden and complete occlusion of the anterior chamber angle by iris tissue (Figure 4.1). The condition is serious. The more common chronic open-angle glaucoma causes no redness of the eye. (See Chapter 3 for a discussion of glaucoma.)

Iritis or Iridocyclitis

Iritis (more strictly iridocyclitis) is an inflammation of the iris alone or of the iris and ciliary body, often manifested by ciliary flush (Figure 4.2). The condition is serious.

Herpes Simplex Keratitis

Herpes simplex keratitis is an infection of the cornea caused by the herpes simplex virus (Figure 4.3). This form of keratitis is common, potentially serious, and can lead to corneal ulceration or scarring. Characteristic dendrites can often be seen in the corneal epithelium.

Conjunctivitis

Conjunctivitis is hyperemia of the conjunctival blood vessels (Figure 4.4). Causes fall into several categories including bacterial, viral, or allergic; exposure to chemical irritants (including eye drops); or mechanical irritation (eg, eyelashes or foreign bodies). Conjunctivitis is common and often not serious.

Episcleritis

Episcleritis is an inflammation (often sectoral) of the episclera, the vascular layer between the conjunctiva and the sclera. The condition is uncommon and has the following features: no discharge, not serious, possibly allergic, and often tender over the inflamed area.

Associated With Soft Contact Lenses

A red eye associated with soft contact lenses can be due to poor fit or inadequate lens hygiene. Symptoms can range from mild conjunctival or superficial corneal irritation to a more serious, vision-threatening infection of the cornea. Referral to an ophthalmologist is advised to interpret the subtle slit-lamp findings.

Scleritis

Scleritis is an inflammation (localized or diffuse) of the sclera (Figure 4.5) that is uncommon, often protracted, and usually accompanied by pain, which may be severe. A violaceous hue of sclera may indicate serious systemic disease such as a collagen vascular disorder.

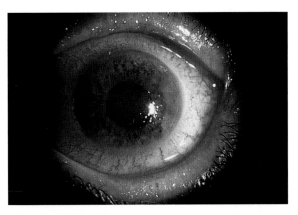

FIGURE 4.1 Acute angle-closure glaucoma. The irregular corneal reflection and hazy cornea suggest edema. The pupil is mid-dilated; the iris appears to be displaced anteriorly, with shallowing of the anterior chamber. These findings plus elevated intraocular pressure are diagnostic of acute angle-closure glaucoma.

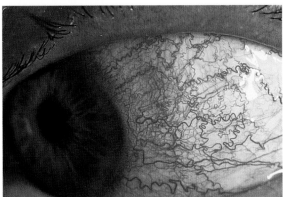

FIGURE 4.2 Ciliary flush. Dilated deep conjunctival and episcleral vessels adjacent and circumferential to the corneal limbus cast a violet hue characteristic of ciliary flush and best seen in natural light.

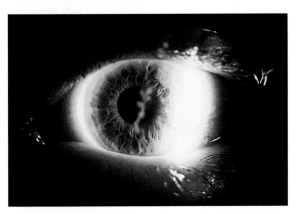

FIGURE 4.3 Herpes simplex keratitis. In the center of the cornea is an irregular, dendritic (branchlike) lesion of the corneal epithelium.

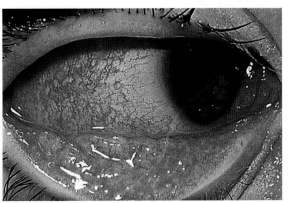

FIGURE 4.4 Conjunctivitis. The hyperemia seen here is produced by a diffuse dilation of the conjunctival blood vessels. The dilation tends to be less intense in the perilimbal region, in contrast to the perilimbal dilation of deeper vessels characteristic of ciliary flush.

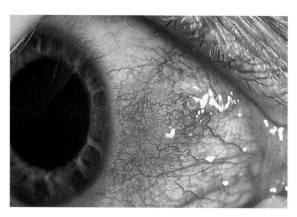

FIGURE 4.5 Scleritis. This localized, raised hyperemic lesion is characteristic of scleritis, which is associated with collagen vascular disorders and rheumatoid diseases. In contrast, episcleritis appears flat, involves more superficial tissue, and is usually not associated with serious systemic disease. The cause of episcleritis may be allergic.

Adnexal Disease

Adnexal disease affects the eyelids, lacrimal apparatus, and orbit and includes dacryocystitis (Figure 4.6), stye, and blepharitis. A red eye can also occur secondary to lid lesions (such as basal cell carcinoma, squamous cell carcinoma, or molluscum contagiosum), thyroid disease, and vascular lesions in the orbit.

Subconjunctival Hemorrhage

A subconjunctival hemorrhage is an accumulation of blood in the potential space between the conjunctiva and the sclera (see Figure 5.10); it is rarely serious.

Pterygium

Pterygium is an abnormal growth consisting of a triangular fold of tissue that advances progressively over the cornea, usually from the nasal side (Figure 4.7). It is usually not serious. Localized conjunctival inflammation may be associated with pterygium. It is associated with ultraviolet exposure and occurs more frequently in tropical climates. Surgical excision is indicated if the pterygium starts to encroach on the visual axis.

Keratoconjunctivitis Sicca

Keratoconjunctivitis sicca, commonly called *dry eye*, is a disorder involving the conjunctiva and sclera resulting from lacrimal deficiency. It is usually not serious.

Abrasions and Foreign Bodies

Hyperemia can occur in response to corneal abrasions or foreign-body injury.

Corneal Ulcerations

Loss of the integrity of the corneal epithelium accompanied with infection or inflammation can result in an ulcer with associated hyperemia. Often the normally clear cornea appears hazy or white in the area of the ulcer. Mucus secretions in the eye (called *mattering*) and pain are common as well as photophobia.

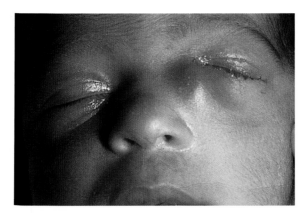

FIGURE 4.6 Dacryocystitis. This obvious, raised erythematous mass represents an acute inflammation of the lacrimal sac, usually secondary to a nasolacrimal duct obstruction. A purulent discharge may be extruded from the lid puncta by massage over the lacrimal sac.

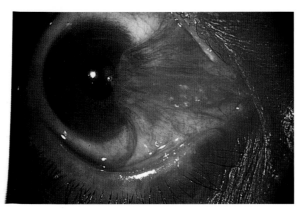

FIGURE 4.7 Pterygium. This wedge-shaped growth of vascularized conjunctiva extends onto the cornea. The initial sign of pterygium may be a localized chronic conjunctivitis.

Secondary to Abnormal Eyelid Function

Bell palsy, thyroid ophthalmopathy, or other conditions can cause ocular exposure and corneal breakdown and may present with a red eye. *Lagophthalmos*, or poor lid closure, is also commonly seen in comatose patients and can result in exposure keratitis, corneal ulceration, and blindness. Eyelids that do not appose the eye well can cause exposure problems and a red eye. An eyelid that turns in toward the eye with the lashes contacting the globe surface can result in pain, photophobia, tearing, and redness of the eye.

HISTORY

When a patient presents with a red eye, taking a thorough history is essential to making the correct diagnosis and initiating appropriate management. Occasionally a red eye may indicate systemic disease; therefore, a complete medical history and review of systems is required.

Additional questions to ask include the following:

- Was the onset sudden? progressive?
- What is the timeline of symptoms? hours or days? intermittent?
- Any family members with red eye recently?
- Is the patient using any over-the-counter or prescription eye medications?
- Is there a history of trauma or out-of-the-ordinary activity recently?

- Has the patient had recent eye surgery? (If so, immediately refer the patient to the surgeon who performed the procedure.)
- Does the patient wear contact lenses? If so, does the patient sleep in the contacts; when were the contacts last changed, and has anything recently changed regarding care of the lens?
- Has the patient had a recent cold or upper respiratory tract infection?
- Has the vision decreased?
- Is there pain? If so, can the patient describe the pain?
- Is there discharge from the involved eye(s)?
- If there is discharge, is it scant or profuse? watery or purulent?
- Is the eye itching?
- Is there light sensitivity?
- Do the symptoms change with environment?
- Has the eye been rubbed or "picked at"?
- Are any other symptoms associated with the red eye?

HOW TO EXAMINE

Nine diagnostic steps are used to evaluate a patient with a red eye:

1. Determine whether the visual acuity is normal or decreased, using a Snellen chart (see Chapter 1).
2. Decide by inspection what pattern of redness is present and whether it is due to subconjunctival hemorrhage, conjunctival hyperemia, ciliary flush, or a combination of these.
3. Detect the presence of conjunctival discharge and categorize it as to amount—profuse or scant—and character—purulent (Figure 4.8), mucopurulent, or serous.
4. Detect opacities of the cornea, including large keratic precipitates (Figure 4.9), corneal edema (Figure 4.10), corneal leukoma (a white opacity caused by scar tissue or corneal infiltrate, Figure 4.11), and irregular corneal reflection (Figure 4.12). Examination is done using a penlight or transilluminator.

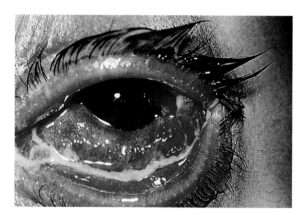

FIGURE 4.8 Purulent conjunctivitis. With the lower lid everted, a creamy-white exudate is visible, highlighted by the conjunctival hyperemia.

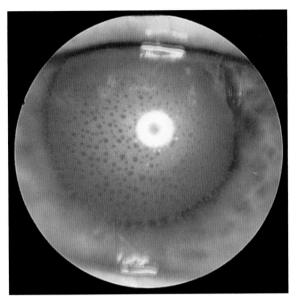

FIGURE 4.9 Large keratic precipitates. Multiple gray-white opacities on the back surface of the cornea are seen against the background of the red reflex. These precipitates can result from chronic iridocyclitis.

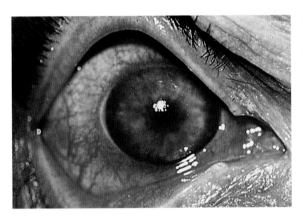

FIGURE 4.10 Corneal edema. In this fiery red eye, the normally sharp corneal reflex is replaced by a diffuse, hazy appearance. Iris details are not as clear as in a healthy eye.

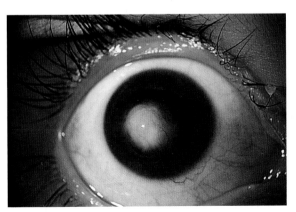

FIGURE 4.11 Corneal leukoma. This dense, white corneal scar represents fibrosis secondary to a previous corneal insult, most frequently trauma or infection. Outside the scar, the cornea is clear. If the scar encroaches on the visual axis, acuity may be impaired.

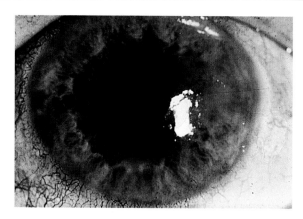

FIGURE 4.12 Irregular corneal reflection. This localized irregularity of the normally sharp corneal light reflection indicates local disruption of the corneal epithelium.

5. Search for disruption of the corneal epithelium by staining the cornea with fluorescein (see Chapter 1).
6. Estimate the depth of the anterior chamber as normal or shallow (see Chapter 1); detect any layered blood or pus, which would indicate either hyphema or hypopyon, respectively. (Compare Figure 4.13, a corneal ulcer with hypopyon, with hyphema, Figure 5.3.)
7. Detect irregularity of the pupils and determine whether one pupil is larger than the other. Observe the reactivity of the pupils to light to determine whether one pupil is more sluggish than the other or is nonreactive (see Chapters 1 and 7).
8. If elevated intraocular pressure is suspected, as in angle-closure glaucoma, and reliable tonometry is available, then measurement of intraocular pressure can help confirm the diagnosis. (Tonometry is omitted when there is an obvious external infection.)
9. Detect the presence of proptosis (Figure 4.14), lid malfunction, or any limitations of eye movement.

HOW TO INTERPRET THE FINDINGS

Although many conditions can cause a red eye, and the associated signs and symptoms of the various disorders overlap to some extent, several signs and symptoms signal danger. The presence of 1 or more of these danger signals should alert the physician that the patient has a disorder requiring an ophthalmologist's attention. Tables 4.1 and 4.2 summarize significant symptoms and signs in the differential diagnosis of a red eye.

SYMPTOMS OF A RED EYE

In the symptoms of a red eye that follow, a red symbol ⚠ by the heading indicates a danger signal.

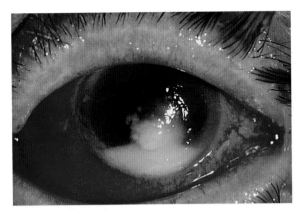

FIGURE 4.13 Corneal ulcer with hypopyon. This inflamed eye shows a white corneal opacity associated with an irregular corneal reflex. In addition, a prominent layering of purulent material appears in the inferior aspect of the anterior chamber, a hypopyon.

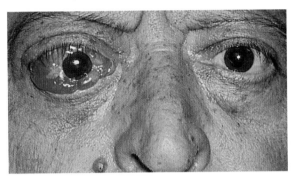

FIGURE 4.14 Chronic proptosis. The right eye of this patient is proptotic, or anteriorly displaced. Marked edema (chemosis) with hyperemia of the conjunctiva is also evident, with tissue prolapse over the lower lid margin. The patient has an orbital tumor.

 Blurred Vision

Blurred vision often indicates serious ocular disease (see "Reduced Visual Acuity" in the following section, "Signs of a Red Eye"). Blurred vision that improves with blinking suggests a discharge or mucus on the ocular surface.

 Severe Pain

Pain may indicate keratitis, ulcer, iridocyclitis, scleritis, or acute glaucoma. Patients with conjunctivitis may complain of a scratchiness or mild irritation but not of severe pain.

⚠ Photophobia

Photophobia is an abnormal sensitivity to light that accompanies iritis, either alone or secondary to corneal inflammation. Patients with conjunctivitis have normal light sensitivity.

 Colored Halos

Rainbow-like fringes or colored halos seen around a point of light are usually a symptom of corneal edema, often resulting from an abrupt rise in intraocular pressure. Therefore, colored halos are a danger signal suggesting acute glaucoma as the cause of a red eye.

TABLE 4.1 Symptoms of a Red Eye

SYMPTOM	REFERRAL ADVISABLE IF PRESENT	ACUTE GLAUCOMA	ACUTE IRIDO-CYCLITIS	KERATITIS	BACTERIAL CONJUNC-TIVITIS	VIRAL CONJUNC-TIVITIS	ALLERGIC CONJUNC-TIVITIS
Blurred vision	Yes	3	1 to 2	3	0	0	0
Pain	Yes	2 to 3	2	2	0	0	0
Photophobia	Yes	1	3	3	0	0	0
Colored halos	Yes	2	0	0	0	0	0
Exudation	No	0	0	0 to 3	3	2	1
Itching	No	0	0	0	0	0	2 to 3

Note: The range of severity of the symptom is indicated by 0 (absent) to 3 (severe).

TABLE 4.2 Signs of a Red Eye

SIGN	REFERRAL ADVISABLE IF PRESENT	ACUTE GLAUCOMA	ACUTE IRIDO-CYCLITIS	KERATITIS	BACTERIAL CONJUNC-TIVITIS	VIRAL CONJUNC-TIVITIS	ALLERGIC CONJUNC-TIVITIS
Ciliary flush	Yes	+	+	+	−	−	−
Conjunctival hyperemia	No	+	+	+	+	+	+
Corneal opacification	Yes	+	−	+	−	+/−	−
Corneal epithelial disruption	Yes	−	−	+	−	+/−	−
Pupillary abnormalities	Yes	+	+	+/−	−	−	−
Shallow anterior chamber	Yes	+	−	−	−	−	−
Elevated intraocular pressure	Yes	+	+/−	−	−	−	−
Proptosis	Yes	−	−	−	−	−	−
Discharge	No	−	−	+/−	+	+	+
Preauricular lymph-node enlargement	No	−	−	−	−	+	−

Note: + = Usually has sign
        − = Does not usually have sign
       +/− = May or may not have sign

Exudation

Exudation, also called *mattering*, is a typical result of conjunctival or eyelid inflammation and does not occur in iridocyclitis or glaucoma. Patients will often complain that their lids are "stuck together" on awakening from sleep. Corneal ulcer is a serious condition that may or may not be accompanied by exudate.

Itching

Although it is a nonspecific symptom, itching usually indicates an allergic conjunctivitis.

SIGNS OF A RED EYE

In the signs of a red eye that follow, a red symbol ⚠ indicates a danger signal.

Reduced Visual Acuity

Reduced visual acuity suggests a serious ocular disease, such as an inflamed cornea, iridocyclitis, or glaucoma. It never occurs in simple conjunctivitis unless there is associated corneal involvement.

Ciliary Flush

Ciliary flush (see Figure 4.2) is an injection of the deep conjunctival and episcleral vessels surrounding the cornea. It is seen most easily in daylight and appears as a faint violaceous ring in which individual vessels are indiscernible to the unaided eye. Ciliary flush is a danger sign often seen in eyes with corneal inflammation, iridocyclitis, or acute glaucoma. Usually, ciliary flush is not present in conjunctivitis.

Conjunctival Hyperemia

Conjunctival hyperemia (see Figure 4.4) is an engorgement of the larger and more superficial bulbar conjunctival vessels. A nonspecific sign, it may be seen in almost any of the conditions causing a red eye.

Corneal Opacification

In a patient with a red eye, corneal opacities always denote disease. These opacities may be detected by direct illumination with a penlight, or they may be seen with a direct ophthalmoscope (with a plus lens in the viewing aperture) outlined against the red fundus reflex. Several types of corneal opacities may occur:

- Keratic precipitates, or cellular deposits on the corneal endothelium, usually too small to be visible but occasionally forming large clumps; these precipitates can result from iritis or from chronic iridocyclitis (see Figure 4.9).
- A diffuse haze obscuring the pupil and iris markings, characteristic of corneal edema (see Figure 4.10) and frequently seen in acute glaucoma.
- Localized opacities due to keratitis or ulcer (see Figure 4.13).

⚠ Corneal Epithelial Disruption

Disruption of the corneal epithelium occurs in corneal inflammations and trauma. It can be detected in 2 ways:

1. Position yourself so that you can observe the reflection from the cornea of a single light source (eg, window, penlight) as the patient moves the eye into various positions. Epithelial disruptions cause distortion and irregularity of the reflection (see Figure 4.12).
2. Apply fluorescein to the eye. Diseased epithelium or areas denuded of epithelium will stain a bright green. (See Figures 1.12 and 1.13 and accompanying text in Chapter 1 for the technique of fluorescein staining.)

⚠ Pupillary Abnormalities

The pupil in an eye with iridocyclitis typically is somewhat smaller than that of the other eye, due to reflex spasm of the iris sphincter muscle. The pupil is also distorted occasionally by posterior synechiae, which are inflammatory adhesions between the lens and the iris. In acute glaucoma, the pupil is usually fixed, mid-dilated (about 5 to 6 mm), and slightly irregular. Conjunctivitis does not affect the pupil.

Shallow Anterior Chamber Depth

In a red eye, a shallow anterior chamber should always suggest the possibility of acute angle-closure glaucoma (see Figure 4.1). Anterior chamber depth can be estimated through side illumination with a penlight. If possible, compare the anterior chamber depth of the red eye with that of the other, unaffected eye. (See Chapter 1 for details on estimating the depth of the anterior chamber.)

⚠ Elevated Intraocular Pressure

Intraocular pressure (IOP) is unaffected by common causes of red eye other than iridocyclitis (IOP often low) and glaucoma (IOP often elevated). Intraocular pressure should be measured when angle-closure glaucoma is suspected. (See Chapter 1 for the use of tonometry to measure IOP.)

Proptosis

Proptosis is a forward displacement of the globe. Sudden proptosis suggests serious orbital or cavernous sinus disease; in children, orbital infection or tumor should be suspected. The most common cause of chronic proptosis is thyroid disease; however, orbital mass lesions also result in proptosis and should be ruled out early in the diagnosis (Figure 4.14). Proptosis may be accompanied by conjunctival hyperemia or limitation of eye movement. Small amounts of proptosis are detected most easily by tilting the chin up and looking from the chin over the maxilla at the relative corneal position.

Discharge

The type of discharge may be an important clue to the cause of a patient's conjunctivitis. Purulent (creamy-white, see Figure 4.8) or mucopurulent (yellowish) exudate suggests a bacterial cause. Serous (watery, clear, or yellow-tinged) discharge suggests a viral cause. Scant, white, stringy discharge sometimes occurs in allergic conjunctivitis and in keratoconjunctivitis sicca, a condition commonly known as *dry eye.*

Preauricular Lymph-Node Enlargement

Enlargement of the lymph node just in front of the auricle is a frequent sign of viral conjunctivitis. Usually, such enlargement does not occur in acute bacterial conjunctivitis. Preauricular node enlargement can be a prominent feature of some unusual varieties of chronic granulomatous conjunctivitis, known collectively as *Parinaud oculoglandular syndrome.* Cat-scratch fever can present with these findings.

ASSOCIATED SYSTEMIC PROBLEMS

The physician should be aware that systemic conditions may include ocular involvement. (See Chapter 8 for additional details.)

Upper Respiratory Tract Infection and Fever

Infection of the upper respiratory tract accompanied by fever may be associated with conjunctivitis, particularly when these symptoms are due to adenovirus type 3 or type 7 (both of which cause pharyngoconjunctival fever). Allergic conjunctivitis may be associated with the seasonal rhinitis of hay fever.

Erythema Multiforme

Erythema multiforme is a serious systemic disorder, possibly an allergic response to medication, which can result in severe conjunctivitis, irreversible conjunctival scarring, and blindness. In erythema multiforme, bull's-eye or target-shaped red lesions are found on the skin. The name Stevens-Johnson syndrome is given to the form of erythema multiforme associated with ocular involvement.

LABORATORY DIAGNOSIS

In practice, most mild cases of conjunctivitis are managed without laboratory assistance. This represents a compromise with ideal management but is justified by the economic waste of obtaining routine smears and cultures in such a common and benign disease. Most clinicians, after making a presumptive clinical diagnosis of bacterial conjunctivitis, proceed directly to broad-spectrum topical ophthalmic antibiotic treatment. Cases of presumed bacterial conjunctivitis that do not improve after 2 days of antibiotic treatment should be referred to an ophthalmologist for confirmation of the diagnosis and appropriate laboratory studies. In addition, in cases of hyperpurulent conjunctivitis, when copious purulent discharge is produced, conjunctival cultures and ophthalmologic consultation are indicated because of a possible gonococcal cause. Gonococcal hyperpurulent conjunctivitis is a serious, potentially blinding disease.

In doubtful cases, smears of exudate or conjunctival scrapings can confirm clinical impressions regarding the type of conjunctivitis. Typical findings include polymorphonuclear cells and bacteria in bacterial conjunctivitis, lymphocytes in viral conjunctivitis, and eosinophils in allergic conjunctivitis. Cultures for bacteria and determinations of antibiotic sensitivity are useful in cases resistant to therapy.

MANAGEMENT OR REFERRAL

The following conditions either require no treatment or may be appropriately treated by a primary care physician. Patients with chronic, unilateral blepharitis should be referred to an ophthalmologist to rule out a malignant process such as sebaceous cell carcinoma or squamous cell carcinoma.

Cases requiring prolonged treatment or those in which the expected response to treatment does not occur promptly should also be referred to an ophthalmologist. (See Table 4.3 for a summary of instructions for patients to follow.)

BLEPHARITIS

Response to the treatment of blepharitis, or inflammation of the eyelid, is often frustratingly slow, and relapses are common. The inflammation of the eyelid can primarily be in the anterior aspect of the lid such as in staphylococcal blepharitis or posterior aspect of the lid as in rosacea blepharitis. Treatment should address the following considerations.

TABLE 4.3 Summary of Patient Instructions for Conditions Related to a Red Eye

CONDITION	PATIENT INSTRUCTION
Blepharitis	Apply warm compresses and eyelid margin scrubs each morning and before bedtime. Apply ointments or take oral medications as prescribed.
Stye and chalazion	Apply warm compresses to the affected eyelid 2 to 4 times daily. Return for further evaluation if the mass fails to disappear after several weeks. Call sooner if the lid mass enlarges, becomes more tender, or begins draining purulent material.
Subconjunctival hemorrhage	Know that without treatment the hemorrhage will resolve in 1 to 2 weeks without any damage to the eye.
Viral conjunctivitis	Apply cool compresses periodically. Use artificial tears if needed. Wash hands frequently and avoid touching eyes and sharing towels. Avoid communal activities as long as discharge is present. Return for referral if symptoms appear to worsen.
Bacterial conjunctivitis	Apply cool compresses periodically and keep lids and lashes free of discharge. Use artificial tears as needed for surface irritation. Apply antibiotic eye drops as prescribed.

Lid Hygiene

Warm compresses (tap water on clean washcloth) can be applied for 3 to 5 minutes, each morning and before bedtime. If lids are oily, follow with lid scrubs using dilute baby shampoo (2 drops shampoo in 2 oz water).

Staphylococcal Infection

Staphylococcal infection (Figure 4.15) may be present. If so, it should be treated with application of appropriate antibiotic ointment (bacitracin or erythromycin) to the lid margin at night for 1 week.

Associated Acne Rosacea/Meibomian Gland Dysfunction

These symptoms should be treated with doxycycline 100 mg twice a day and tapered to once a day for 2 months or longer. Artificial tears may be applied 4 to 8 times a day as needed for symptoms of dryness.

Scalp Seborrhea

Treatment with antidandruff shampoos can improve symptoms of seborrheic blepharitis (Figure 4.16).

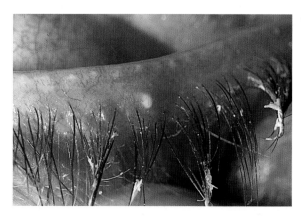

FIGURE 4.15 Staphylococcal blepharitis. Chronic staphylococcal lid infection produces inflamed, swollen lids that may ulcerate. The oily discharge binds the lashes and sometimes condenses to form a collarette around a lash.

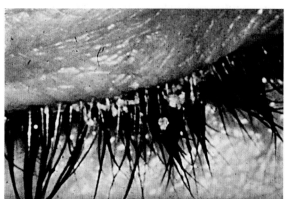

FIGURE 4.16 Seborrheic blepharitis. The dry, flaky lashes and red lid margins seen here are characteristic of seborrheic blepharitis.

Contact Dermatitis

Contact dermatitis (Figure 4.17) can masquerade as blepharitis. A careful history of the lid redness associated with application of medication helps make the diagnosis. For example, the glaucoma medication brimonidine can produce a red eye with erythematous, swollen lids that have a dry "leathery" texture. Any ocular medication or cosmetics can be associated with similar clinical findings. Discontinuing the offending product should result in improvement in symptoms within 48 hours, but healing may take up to 2 weeks.

STYE AND CHALAZION

A stye, or *hordeolum*, is an acute, usually sterile, inflammation of the glands or hair follicles in the eyelid. Hordeola can be categorized as external or internal, according to where the inflammation is located in the lid (Figures 4.18 and 4.19). A chalazion is a chronic inflammation of a meibomian gland in the eyelid that may develop spontaneously or may follow a hordeolum (Figure 4.20). A persistent or recurring lid mass should undergo biopsy because it may be a rare meibomian gland carcinoma or squamous cell carcinoma of the lid rather than a benign chalazion.

The mainstays of treatment are the following:

- Apply warm compresses to the eyelid 4 times a day for 3 to 5 minutes.
- Massage the lid and lash line to encourage the glands to open up and drain.
- Apply topical ocular antibiotic ointment to the lash line and over the area if there is tenderness and infection is suspected. Rarely, oral antibiotics may be indicated if there is a secondary bacterial infection.
- Refer the patient for incision and curettage of the lesion if there is no resolution in 3 to 4 weeks.

SUBCONJUNCTIVAL HEMORRHAGE

In the absence of blunt trauma, hemorrhage into the subconjunctiva, the potential space between the conjunctiva and the sclera, requires no treatment and, unless recurrent, no evaluation (see Figure 5.10). Causes include a sudden increase in ocular venous pressure, such as occurs with coughing, sneezing, vomiting, or vigorous rubbing of the eye. Many subconjunctival hemorrhages occur during sleep. If recurrent, an underlying bleeding disorder should be considered. Blood pressure should be measured, as marked elevation can result in subconjunctival hemorrhage.

CONJUNCTIVITIS

There is no specific medicinal treatment for viral conjunctivitis, although patients should be instructed in proper precautions to prevent contagion. Here are some treatments often recommended:

- Apply cool compresses periodically throughout the day.
- Use artificial tear drops if irritation occurs.

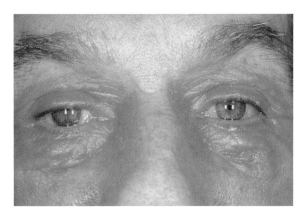

FIGURE 4.17 Contact dermatitis. Allergic contact dermatitis shown here is secondary to topical ophthalmic medication. (Reprinted from *Basic and Clinical Science Course,* Section 8: External Disease and Cornea. San Francisco, CA: American Academy of Ophthalmology; 2009–2010:206.)

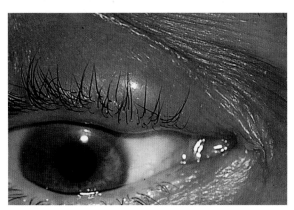

FIGURE 4.18 External hordeolum. This large, acute swelling, which is red and painful, involves the hair follicles or associated glands of Zeis or Moll and points toward the skin.

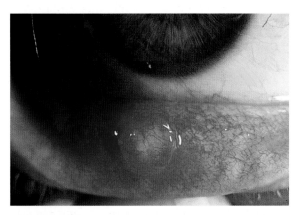

FIGURE 4.19 Internal hordeolum. An acute infection of a meibomian gland produces a swelling directed internally toward the conjunctiva. This figure demonstrates a discrete, circumscribed area of inflammation highlighted by a hyperemic conjunctiva.

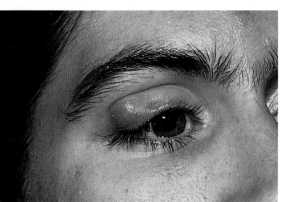

FIGURE 4.20 Chalazion. This large, nontender lid mass is a chronic granulomatous inflammation of a meibomian gland.

- Apply antibiotic eye drops 4 to 6 times a day if bacterial infection is suspected (sulfacetamide, gentamicin, or any broad-spectrum topical antibiotic).
- Minimize spread to other family members and co-workers (eg, washing hands after touching eye secretions, no sharing of towels).

It cannot be emphasized too strongly that corticosteroids have limited use in treatment of infectious conjunctivitis. Eye drops containing a combination of antibiotics and corticosteroids should be used only under the close observation of an ophthalmologist.

THERAPEUTIC WARNINGS

Because of possible serious health risks, caution is required in the use of the following therapeutic agents.

Topical Anesthetics

Topical anesthetics should never be prescribed for prolonged analgesia in ocular inflammations and injuries for 3 reasons:

- Topical anesthetics inhibit growth and healing of the corneal epithelium.
- Although rare, severe allergic reaction may result from instillation of topical anesthetics.
- Corneal anesthesia eliminates the protective blink reflex, exposing the cornea to dehydration, injury, and infection.

Topical Corticosteroids

Topical corticosteroids have 3 potentially serious ocular side effects:

- Both herpes simplex keratitis (see Figure 4.3) and fungal keratitis are markedly potentiated by corticosteroids. Corticosteroids may mask symptoms of inflammation, making the patient "feel" better, while the cornea may be melting away or even perforating.
- Prolonged use of corticosteroids, either locally or systemically, often leads to cataract formation.
- Local application of corticosteroids for 2 to 6 weeks may cause an elevation of intraocular pressure in approximately one-third of the population. The pressure rise may be severe in a small percentage of cases. Optic nerve damage and permanent loss of vision can occur. The combination of a corticosteroid and an antibiotic carries the same risk. Topical corticosteroids alone or in combination with antibiotics should not be administered to the eye by a primary care physician. They can be very helpful when used under the close supervision of an ophthalmologist.

POINTS TO REMEMBER

- If visual acuity is acutely and significantly reduced, a diagnosis of conjunctivitis is extremely unlikely.
- Fluorescein should always be instilled in a red eye to test for integrity of the corneal epithelium.
- A pupillary inequality in a patient with red eye(s) is a danger signal for serious ocular disease.
- If the patient wears soft contact lenses, referral to an ophthalmologist is advised because differentiation between mild and severe complications of contact lens wear requires experienced interpretation of slit-lamp findings.
- In obtaining a history for the red eye, the examiner should document all medications applied in and around the eye and then consider them as the potential source of the red eye.

SAMPLE PROBLEMS

1. A 23-year-old teacher complains that her right eye is red and irritated. You note moderate injection of the larger conjunctival vessels, watery discharge, and a palpable preauricular lymph node.

   A. From this information alone, what tentative diagnosis would you make?

   Answer: The conjunctival injection and discharge suggest conjunctivitis. The serous nature of the discharge, plus the preauricular adenopathy, indicate that she has viral conjunctivitis.

   B. Again based on the above information, which of the following symptoms or facts might be elicited by careful history-taking?

   a. Blurred vision
   b. Sore throat
   c. Exposure to children with colds
   d. Itching

   Answer: b and c. Sore throat often accompanies viral conjunctivitis; in such cases, a history of exposure to other individuals with upper respiratory tract infections can often be elicited. Blurred vision, a danger signal of serious ocular disease, is not a feature of simple conjunctivitis. Itching is a symptom of allergic, not viral, conjunctivitis.

   C. Management consists of which of the following?

   a. Corticosteroid eyed drops
   b. Broad-spectrum antibiotic eye drops
   c. Referral to an ophthalmologist
   d. Instruction to the patient to use cool compresses and stay home from school until the redness resolves

Answer: d. Because the disease is contagious, the patient should be instructed to remain home from work. There is no specific medicinal treatment for viral conjunctivitis. Corticosteroids may be used only under the close supervision of an ophthalmologist.

2. A young woman complains of a red eye and associated pain above the eye. The patient's mother has chronic open-angle glaucoma and the patient wants to know whether she has the same thing. The patient describes several bouts of having a red, painful, left eye that is relieved by sleeping.

   A. You notice an irregular pupil in addition to the injection of her left eye. This would be more consistent with which of the following?

      a. Angle-closure glaucoma
      b. Iridocyclitis
      c. Conjunctivitis
      d. Keratitis sicca
      e. Chronic open-angle glaucoma

   Answer: a and b. Both angle-closure glaucoma and iridocyclitis can have an irregular pupil, pain, and redness. Anterior surface problems like conjunctivitis and keratitis sicca (dry eye) should not result in an irregular pupil. Chronic open-angle glaucoma does not present with a red, inflamed eye. It does not give an irregular pupil.

   B. On further questioning, the patient describes seeing colored halos around lights. What is the most likely diagnosis of those listed in part A, above?

   Answer: a. Angle-closure glaucoma

3. A 45-year-old man reports a 2-day history of redness, severe pain, and photophobia of his left eye. He denies any trauma to the eye.

   A. Which of the following signs convince you the patient does not have conjunctivitis?

      a. Visual acuity of 20/200
      b. Conjunctival injection
      c. Ciliary flush
      d. Serous discharge

   Answer: a and c. Reduced visual acuity, as well as ciliary flush, often signals ocular disease more serious than conjunctivitis.

   B. You note that there is staining of the cornea in a branching pattern. What is the most likely diagnosis?

   Answer: Keratitis, possibly herpetic

C. In possible herpetic keratitis, what would your management be?

    a. A telephone request to an ophthalmologist for immediate examination

    b. Corticosteroid drops to decrease inflammation and follow-up with an ophthalmologist in 3 to 5 days

    c. An oral antiviral like acyclovir and follow-up in a week

Answer: a. Herpetic keratitis is a serious infection and can be vision threatening. Immediate referral is indicated to decrease the potential scarring and permanent loss of vision. Steroid drops are never indicated in a patient with active disease and epithelial staining. Steroid drops can cause corneal melting and possible perforation of the eye.

4. A 38-year-old woman complains of a 3-day history of a red, tender right eyelid. Physical examination reveals a tender nodule of the right lower eyelid with minimal injection of the inferior conjunctiva.

A. Which of the following would constitute appropriate management by the primary care physician? (More than 1 course of action may be possible.)

    a. Warm compresses

    b. Broad-spectrum systemic antibiotics

    c. Topical antibiotics

    d. Immediate surgical incision and drainage to prevent cellulitis

Answer: a and c. The patient has a stye. Because she has only had symptoms for 3 days and the lesion is tender to touch, she would benefit from warm compresses. Topical antibiotic ointment might benefit a small percentage of patients. Incision and drainage is indicated only when lesions do not resolve spontaneously or with medical therapy. Usually surgical intervention occurs only after the lesion has been present for several weeks. Systemic antibiotics are not indicated.

B. If the patient reports she has had numerous nodules in this same area over the last 5 years, how should the primary care physician change the management plan?

Answer: A persistent or recurring lid mass should undergo biopsy to rule out an eyelid malignancy. Referral to an ophthalmologist is indicated.

5. An 88-year-old nursing home patient has had red, irritated eyes for months. She feels like she has "sand in her eyes" all the time. On examination, all 4 eyelid margins are inflamed and edematous with debris on the lashes.

A. What is the most likely diagnosis?

Answer: Blepharitis

B. Treatment would consist of which of the following?

  a. Immediate referral to an ophthalmologist
  b. Cleansing of the eyelids daily
  c. Antibiotic ointment to alleviate any staphylococcal infection

Answer: b and c. Blepharitis is a chronic, often relapsing, inflammation of the eyelids that can irritate the eyes. A low-grade bacterial infection may be involved. It is not an ophthalmologic emergency and treatment is long-term daily lid hygiene. For difficult cases, an appointment with an ophthalmologist is indicated.

6. A 65-year-old man with history of a recent bronchitis awoke this morning with a red eye and has no other symptoms. He has no significant medical problems.

  A. On examination, the patient has a sector of the eye that is solid red without injection of the conjunctival vessels. What is the most likely diagnosis?

  a. Scleritis
  b. Subconjunctival hemorrhage
  c. Early viral conjunctivitis
  d. Pterygium

  Answer: b. A subconjunctival hemorrhage is in the potential space between the conjunctiva and sclera. The conjunctival and deeper vessels are not injected or inflamed as in conjunctivitis or scleritis. Scleritis can appear in a sector pattern, but is usually associated with pain or tenderness. A pterygium forms due to chronic UV exposure and presents over years, not overnight.

  B. The recent bronchitis may be associated with the subconjunctival hemorrhage in what way?

  Answer: The patient may have had an episode of coughing during the night, resulting in a sudden increase in ocular venous pressure that can cause a subconjunctival hemorrhage. Aggressive eye rubbing can cause a subconjunctival hemorrhage, but more commonly it occurs without any identifiable precipitating event. Patients with subconjunctival hemorrhage should be questioned about easy bruising, and the blood pressure should be checked.

7. You are called to a nursing home to see an 84-year-old woman with a red, painful eye. When you examine her, you note that visual acuity is decreased in the affected eye and that the lower lid appears to be turning in toward the eye.

  A. The cornea appears white and hazy inferiorly, and the patient is complaining of photophobia. What is the most likely diagnosis?

  a. Conjunctivitis
  b. Corneal ulcer
  c. Old corneal scar
  d. Scleritis

Answer: b. Corneal ulcer. A white and hazy cornea represents either active inflammation or a scar. Pain and photophobia are associated with an active process, not an old corneal scar. Conjunctivitis and scleritis are inflammatory disorders of other parts of the eye, not the cornea.

B. What is the most likely underlying cause of the corneal problem in this patient?

   a. The eyelid and lashes scraping the cornea with resulting ulceration and infection
   b. Cat-scratch fever
   c. Chronic open-angle glaucoma

Answer: a. Entropion is the inward turning of the eyelid in which the lashes may abrade the cornea and cause an epithelial defect. Bacteria can then infect the exposed corneal stroma with resulting inflammation and opacity of the normally clear cornea. Inferior corneal ulceration implicates the lower lid as the source of the ulcer. Cat-scratch fever does not usually cause a corneal ulcer, and chronic open-angle glaucoma is not associated with a red eye.

ANNOTATED RESOURCES

Albert DM, Jakobiec FA, eds. *Principles and Practice of Ophthalmology: Clinical Practice.* 3rd ed. Philadelphia, PA: WB Saunders Co; 2008. This comprehensive text includes information relevant to conditions presenting with red eye.

Newell FW. *Ophthalmology: Principles and Concepts.* 8th ed. St Louis, MO: CV Mosby Co; 1996. This comprehensive text includes detailed discussions of diseases of the conjunctiva and cornea.

Tasman W, Jaeger EA, eds. *Duane's Ophthalmology.* CD-ROM. 15th ed. Philadelphia, PA: Lippincott Williams & Wilkins; 2009. This comprehensive work includes discussions of various forms of conjunctivitis and anterior uveitis. Updated, comprehensive discussions of various forms of conjunctivitis are found in chapters 4–9A and of anterior uveitis in chapters 39–42.

Trobe JD. *The Physician's Guide to Eye Care.* 3rd ed. San Francisco, CA: American Academy of Ophthalmology; 2006. A brief but comprehensive resource covering the principal clinical ophthalmic problems that nonophthalmologist physicians are likely to encounter, organized for practical use by practitioners.

Ocular and Orbital Injuries

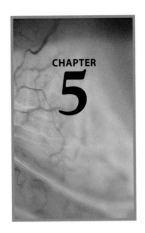

OBJECTIVES

As a primary care physician, you should be able to evaluate the common ocular or orbital injuries and to determine whether or not the problem requires the prompt attention of an ophthalmologist. In situations of true ocular emergency, such as chemical burns, you should be able to institute therapy when necessary. To achieve these objectives, you should learn to

> ➤ Recognize which problems are emergent or urgent and deal with them accordingly
> ➤ Obtain the salient historical facts
> ➤ Examine the traumatized eye
> ➤ Record the visual acuity as accurately as possible
> ➤ Competently manage or appropriately refer the most common injuries

RELEVANCE

One day, whether in your own home or yard or while on duty in the emergency center, you will be confronted with an unexpected ocular injury. Your skill in dealing with major eye injuries can mean the difference between preservation and loss of a patient's vision. The purpose of this chapter is to assist in developing confidence when approaching minor or major eye injuries; it will further your competence in acquiring the basic techniques and knowledge necessary to assess and initiate treatment of the eye and its surrounding structures.

BASIC INFORMATION

This section introduces ocular and periocular anatomy and helps you identify emerging or urgent ocular problems.

ANATOMY AND FUNCTION

The following lists structures of the eye, their role, and how they might be impacted by injury.

Bony Orbit

- The orbit is the bony, concave cavity in the skull housing the globe, extraocular muscles, and blood vessels and nerves of the eye (Figure 5.1).
- The rim of the orbit protects the globe from impact with large objects.
- A rim fracture usually causes no decrease in ocular or visual function.
- The very thin orbital floor (consisting of the maxillary, palatine, and zygomatic bones) may "blow out" into the maxillary sinus from blunt impact to the orbit, for instance, from a fist or tennis ball. Orbital contents, including the inferior rectus and inferior oblique muscles, may become trapped, restricting vertical eye movement and causing double vision (termed *diplopia*). An orbital floor fracture is often associated with decreased sensation or numbness of the cheek and teeth on the ipsilateral side. In medial wall and floor fractures, bleeding from the nose may occur acutely after the injury.
- A medial fracture of the thin ethmoid bone may be associated with subcutaneous emphysema of the eyelids. The patient with an acute orbital fracture should avoid blowing the nose.
- A fracture at or near the optic canal, through which the optic nerve and ophthalmic artery pass, may cause damage to the optic nerve or the vessels that supply it (traumatic optic neuropathy), with resulting visual loss.

Eyelids

- The lids close reflexively when the eyes are threatened.
- The act of blinking rewets the cornea through constant surface contact and tear production.

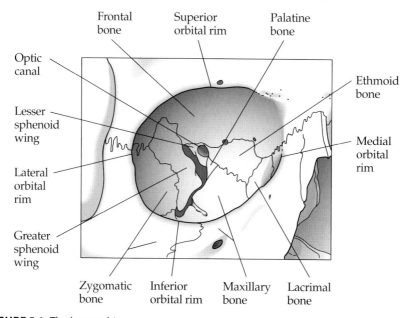

FIGURE 5.1 The bony orbit.

- In the case of a facial nerve palsy, the globe may be exposed to drying or other injury.
- Lid margins must be intact to ensure proper lid closure and tear drainage.

Lacrimal Apparatus

- Tear drainage occurs at the medial aspect of the lids, primarily through the lower lacrimal punctum, and continues through the canaliculi to the lacrimal sac, and via the nasolacrimal duct to the nose (Figure 1.2).
- Failure to recognize and properly repair a canalicular laceration can result in chronic tearing (epiphora).

Conjunctiva and Cornea

- The corneal epithelium usually heals quickly following an abrasion.
- Small lacerations of the conjunctiva heal quickly and, consequently, may conceal a penetrating injury of the globe.

Anterior Chamber

- The aqueous humor often escapes in penetrating corneal injuries, sometimes resulting in a shallow or flat anterior chamber (see Figure 1.1).

Iris and Ciliary Body

- Following laceration or perforation of the cornea or limbus, the iris may prolapse into the wound (see Figure 5.2), resulting in an irregular pupil.
- Blunt trauma to the eyeball may produce iritis, resulting in pain, redness, photophobia, and a small pupil (miosis).
- Contusions may deform the pupil by tearing the iris root or by notching the pupillary margin.
- Contusions may result in tearing of small vessels in the anterior chamber angle, causing hemorrhage into the anterior chamber (hyphema, Figure 5.3). A hyphema is generally the result of trauma and usually resolves spontaneously in 3 to 5 days.

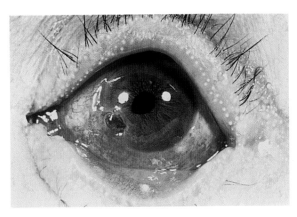

FIGURE 5.2 Corneal perforation with iris prolapse. Slight distortion of the pupil, irregularity of the corneal reflection, and a knuckle of soft, brown tissue at the limbus indicate a corneal perforation through which the iris has prolapsed.

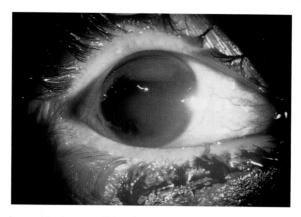

FIGURE 5.3 Hyphema. Hyphema, or blood in the anterior chamber, can result from a tear in peripheral iris vessels and is a potentially serious complication of blunt ocular trauma. Most hyphemas can be readily identified by careful penlight inspection. (Reprinted from "Eye Trauma and Emergencies." In: *Eye Care Skills: Presentations for Physicians and Other Health Care Professionals,* v3.0. San Francisco, CA: American Academy of Ophthalmology; 2009.)

Lens

- Injuries to the lens usually proceed to cataract formation.
- Blunt trauma to the globe can cause a partial dislocation (subluxation) of the lens (Figure 5.4).

Vitreous Humor

- Loss of transparency may be observed in the presence of hemorrhage, inflammation, or infection.

Retina

- The retina is protected externally by the sclera (a tough outer layer) and the choroid (an underlying vascular layer, see Figure 1.1).
- The retina is thin and vulnerable. If penetrated by a foreign body, retinal detachment may occur. (See discussion and Figure 2.2 in Chapter 2.)
- Retinal hemorrhage may develop as a result of direct or indirect trauma.

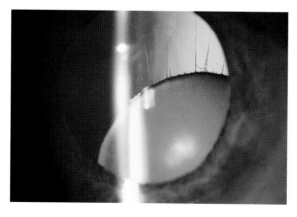

FIGURE 5.4 Subluxated lens. Light reflected off the fundus and back through a dilated pupil silhouettes the edge of a subluxated lens with stretched zonular fibers. Ordinarily, the edge of the lens is not visible even if the pupil is widely dilated.

- The retina turns white when edematous.
- Macular damage will reduce visual acuity without producing complete blindness.

WHEN TO EXAMINE

Most ocular injuries present with obvious redness and pain. However, not all injuries provide such obvious warning signs. For example, a sharp perforation may produce minimal redness and escape attention. The examiner should be especially alert to perforating injuries caused by small projectiles resulting from "striking metal on metal." If there is a history of metal striking metal with something hitting the eye, the patient should be referred to an ophthalmologist for evaluation even if the vision is normal and the eye looks quiet. An intraocular foreign body (Figure 5.5) produces no pain because the lens, retina, and vitreous have no nerve endings to conduct sensations of pain.

If damage to the posterior segment is suspected, including retinal detachment or intraocular foreign body, referral to an ophthalmologist is indicated. The ophthalmologist's examination of the fundus will be facilitated if you do not use ointment in the eye.

HOW TO EXAMINE

When a patient presents with an eye injury, the physician should obtain the patient's history, if possible, and perform a complete examination of the eyes and surrounding structures. This should include visual acuity testing, external examination, assessment of the pupils and eye movements, and ophthalmoscopy. Two sample examinations are in Tables 5.1 and 5.2.

HISTORY

In the evaluation of ocular injuries, it is important to document the type of traumatic event as well as the time of onset and the nature of the symptoms. Specific historical information to obtain includes the time, place, and type of injury (eg, blunt or sharp trauma; acid or alkali burn) and the patient's history of eye

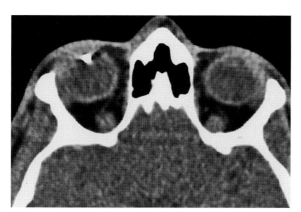

FIGURE 5.5 CT scan of foreign body. A small, radiopaque intraocular foreign body is visible in the anterior segment of the eye.

TABLE 5.1 Sample Examination: Foreign-Body Sensation

AREA	NOTES
History	
Type of injury, time, and place	Foreign-body sensation, 3:15 am, seen in emergency center.
Pertinent chain of events; is trauma centered in OD, OS, or OU?	At about 2:45 am, patient awoke with severe foreign-body sensation OU.
Subjective visual loss, if any, and amount of visual decrease; associated complaints, symptoms	No injury, although admits to using sunlamp to tan face for 20 minutes previous evening. Now unable to open eyes, which aggravates burning foreign-body sensation. Unable to see well but uncertain about degree of visual loss.
Was vision normal prior to injury?	Patient states vision has been normal until now.
Examination	
Best correctable VA for both eyes (ie, with glasses if available, with pinhole if necessary)	Unable to cooperate until 1 drop topical anesthetic (proparacaine 0.5%) administered OU VA: OD 20/25; OS 20/20
Appearance and function of:	
Bony orbit and lids	Bony orbit intact Marked eyelid spasm until anesthetic drops given
Cornea and conjunctiva	Cornea stains irregularly with fluorescein Conjunctival injection OU, pronounced near limbus
Media (aqueous, lens, vitreous)	Media clear on gross inspection
Diagnosis	Ultraviolet conjunctival and corneal injury
Management	Cycloplegic drops, antibiotic ointment, and possibly a pressure dressing. Because these injuries are often bilateral, patch only the worse eye—it is difficult for the patient to function with both eyes patched. A prescription for oral analgesic may be indicated.

conditions, drug allergies, and tetanus immunization. Maintain a high level of suspicion for an open (punctured) globe based on the mechanism of trauma. A history of pounding metal on metal, the patient's statement that something was "pulled out of the eye," or blunt ocular trauma in a patient who has undergone past eye surgery are suggestive of more severe injury. As in any trauma situation, you should not delay prompt treatment to obtain a detailed history if an obvious injury is present, such as a chemical burn.

After significant trauma has occurred, the patient may be unconscious or unable to answer questions. In this case, the physician can question whoever accompanied the patient for as much historical information as possible, but must be prepared to assess the injury and proceed with treatment or referral in the absence of adequate historical information.

TABLE 5.2 Sample Examination: Double Vision

AREA	NOTES
History	
Approximate onset of symptoms	A 16-year-old boy complains that he awoke 2 days ago with a feeling of fullness OS.
Type of symptoms, frequency, regularity	Later, he noted vertical double vision when looking straight up, up and right, and up and left; no double vision when looking straight ahead. No other problem except mild aching when looking up. Hit by knee in left eye in wrestling class 3 days earlier.
Increasing or decreasing severity?	Symptoms unchanged since first noted.
Examination	
Ocular findings	Perform complete eye examination, with particular attention to testing extraocular muscles. Rule out possible damage to the globe. Patient unable to elevate left eye beyond primary gaze. Globe examination unremarkable except for localized subconjunctival hemorrhage. Visual acuity normal.
X-rays	Obtain Waters view, which reveals opacification of the maxillary antrum and downward herniation of orbital structures. CT scan more clearly delineates fracture of orbital floor.
Diagnosis	Blowout fracture left orbit with muscle entrapment.
Management	Refer to an ophthalmologist semiurgently for evaluation and consideration of surgical repair. Start oral antibiotics like cephalexin to prevent possible orbital cellulitis from sinus bacteria, and ask the patient to avoid blowing his nose.

VISUAL ACUITY TESTING

Visual acuity should be recorded as specifically as possible. Refer to Chapter 1 for detailed instructions on assessing visual acuity, including use of the Snellen eye chart. If a Snellen chart is unavailable, determine the patient's ability to read available print material and record the type of print used (eg, newspaper, telephone book) and the distance at which it was read. Note in particular whether vision is equal in both eyes. If vision is below reading level, determine the patient's ability to count fingers, perceive hand motions, or respond to light.

EXTERNAL EXAMINATION

An examination of the external structures of the eye may include palpation, penlight inspection, lid eversion, fluorescein staining, and topical anesthesia. Palpation of the orbital rims should be performed if a blunt injury or fracture is suspected. A penlight is used to inspect the eye for signs of perforation, such as reduced depth of the anterior chamber or iris prolapse (see Figure 5.2). Hyphema (see Figure 5.3) may be present without perforation and, in fact, often accompanies blunt injury. Lid eversion (retraction and eversion of the upper and lower eyelids) will facilitate inspection for a foreign body or chemical burn.

Do not manipulate the eyelids if you suspect a penetrating injury of the globe.

If the patient has a foreign-body sensation or if there is a history of blunt or sharp injury, fluorescein is used to stain the cornea to identify any corneal epithelial defects. (See Chapter 1 for the technique of fluorescein staining.)

Eye drops can be used to provide topical anesthesia, especially to relieve foreign-body sensation or discomfort due to radiant energy burns or prolonged wear of contact lenses. Use of 1 drop of proparacaine hydrochloride 0.5% provides almost instantaneous pain relief and allows you to proceed with an adequate evaluation, including determination of visual acuity, which would otherwise be impossible due to discomfort. Do not prescribe or distribute samples of anesthetic drops or ointment because prolonged use can result in corneal ulceration.

PUPILLARY REACTIONS

Always check pupillary reactions in trauma cases. Diminished direct pupillary reaction to light with an intact consensual response (a relative afferent pupillary defect) may indicate an optic nerve injury (see Chapter 7).

OCULAR MOTILITY TESTING

Movement of the eye may be generally restricted in the case of orbital hematoma. If there is a history of blunt trauma, vertical restriction combined with vertical diplopia should make you suspect a blowout fracture. If limitation of eye movements is accompanied by proptosis, auscultate the head and eye for a bruit, which would be suggestive of a carotid–cavernous sinus fistula.

To avoid extrusion of intraocular contents, do not perform motility testing in suspected globe laceration.

OPHTHALMOSCOPY

If the fundus is visible, look for edema, retinal hemorrhages, retinal detachment, and, if penetration is suspected, a foreign body. In the event of a positive finding or the suspicion of a penetrating injury or foreign body, refer the patient to an ophthalmologist immediately.

The normal red reflex from the fundus is evenly colored and not interrupted by shadows (see Figure 1.14). If the red reflex is absent, immediate referral to an ophthalmologist is indicated. Absence of the red reflex may be due to hyphema, cataract from acute swelling of the lens, or vitreous hemorrhage. Hyphema is visible on external examination with a penlight, whereas the detection of cataract and vitreous hemorrhage requires assessment with an ophthalmoscope.

Pupillary dilation to permit evaluation of the fundus should be routine. The only general exceptions to this rule would be in patients with head trauma where pupillary signs might be important for neurologic evaluation and patients whose shallow anterior chamber predisposes them to narrow-angle glaucoma.

RADIOLOGIC STUDIES

Radiologic evaluation is suggested if there is any question of facial or orbital fracture or of ocular or orbital foreign body. A CT scan can often provide additional useful detail. MRI should not be ordered if a metallic foreign body is suspected, because the metal may heat, vibrate, or move during the scan, resulting in additional intraocular injury.

MANAGEMENT OR REFERRAL

The primary care physician may not be able to provide definitive care for each of the following entities, but should be able to initiate treatment in every case.

TRUE EMERGENCY

Therapy must be instituted within minutes. A chemical burn of the conjunctiva and cornea represents one of the true ocular emergencies. An alkali burn (Figure 5.6) usually results in greater damage to the eye than an acid burn, because alkali compounds (eg, lye, anhydrous ammonia) penetrate ocular tissues more rapidly. All chemical burns require immediate and profuse irrigation, followed by referral to an ophthalmologist.

URGENT SITUATION

Urgent situations require therapy to be instituted within a few hours. The following list describes common urgent ocular situations and appropriate actions to take for each.

Penetrating Injuries of the Globe

Penetrating injuries of the globe, whether actual or suspected, necessitate the protection of an eye shield. Neither a patch nor an ointment is advisable. The patient should be prevented from eating or drinking anything in anticipation of surgical intervention. An x-ray or CT scan of the orbit should be ordered to rule out radiopaque foreign bodies (see Figure 5.5). Referral to an ophthalmologist is indicated.

Conjunctival or Corneal Foreign Bodies

Conjunctival or corneal foreign bodies (Figures 5.7 and 5.8) require topical anesthesia followed by removal of the object with either vigorous irrigation or a cotton-tipped applicator. (See "Foreign-Body Removal" under "Treatment Skills" later in this chapter for specific instructions.)

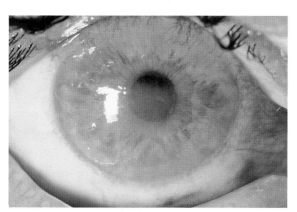

FIGURE 5.6 Alkali burn. Blanching of the conjunctiva and a large corneal epithelial defect, demonstrated by application of fluorescein, indicate a relatively serious injury.

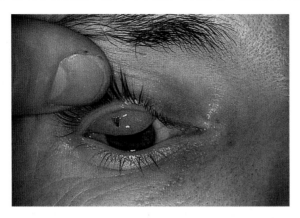

FIGURE 5.7 Conjunctival foreign body. A foreign body often lodges under the edge of the upper eyelid. As this figure shows, the foreign body is easily seen and removed upon eversion of the eyelid.

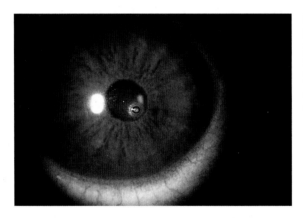

FIGURE 5.8 Corneal foreign body. Visible here is a small piece of iron embedded in the surface of the cornea. Surrounding the iron are a ring of rust and grayish corneal edema.

For corneal abrasions, take the following steps:

1. Anesthetize with proparacaine 0.5%.
2. Perform a gross examination.
3. Stain with fluorescein to enhance the view. (For a depiction of a fluorescein stain delineating a corneal abrasion, see Figures 1.12 and 1.13.)
4. Instill ocular antibiotic drops or ointment; instill short-acting cycloplegic (tropicamide 1% or cyclopentolate 1%) drops for the relief of pain as indicated.
5. Some physicians apply a pressure patch to maintain lid closure for 24 hours, although others feel that abrasions less than 10 mm in diameter heal better and more quickly without a pressure patch. No patch should be applied if the abrasion is associated with contact lens wear.
6. Refer severe cases to an ophthalmologist.

Hyphema

Hyphema requires immediate referral to an ophthalmologist. Elevation of intraocular pressure may necessitate medical or surgical intervention. Also, the hyphema may be a sign of globe rupture or a more serious ocular injury such as dislocated lens or retinal detachment.

Lid Laceration

A lid laceration can be sutured if not deep and neither the lid margin nor the canaliculi are involved; otherwise, refer to an ophthalmologist. (The lid laceration shown in Figure 5.9 would require referral because it is full-thickness and involves the lid margin. There is also a possibility of canalicular involvement because the laceration is close to the medial canthus.)

Radiant Energy Burns

Radiant energy burns, such as welder's burn or snow blindness, require topical anesthesia, examination, topical antibiotic and cycloplegic agents, and possibly patching. Since these injuries are often bilateral, it is difficult for the patient to function with both eyes patched. Many patients prefer simply closing the eyes. The corneal epithelium regenerates quickly, and after several hours the pain is much less intense. (See Chapter 9 for information about instilling ocular medications.)

Traumatic Optic Neuropathy

Traumatic optic neuropathy, although uncommon, should always be considered in patients with cranial or maxillofacial trauma. Patients present with a history of facial or frontal trauma, usually with unilateral decreased vision and a relative afferent pupillary defect, but further examination reveals no clear ocular origin. High-resolution CT imaging of the orbital apex, optic canal, and cavernous sinus is essential if traumatic optic neuropathy is suspected. Patients may benefit from intravenous high-dose methylprednisolone if given in the first 8 hours after initial injury. If a patient is suspected of having traumatic optic neuropathy, a prompt referral to an ophthalmologist is indicated.

SEMIURGENT CONDITION

Refer patients with semiurgent conditions to an ophthalmologist within 1 to 2 days. An orbital fracture falls in this category. Subconjunctival hemorrhage (Figure 5.10) in the presence of blunt trauma is also a semiurgent condition, unless a globe rupture or intraocular hemorrhage is suspected, in which case urgent referral to an ophthalmologist is indicated.

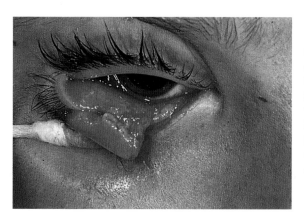

FIGURE 5.9 Full-thickness lid laceration. The lower eyelid is partially everted with the applicator stick, revealing an irregular laceration of the lid margin, orbicularis muscle, tarsal plate, and conjunctiva. Note the proximity of the laceration to the medial canthus, indicating possible canalicular involvement.

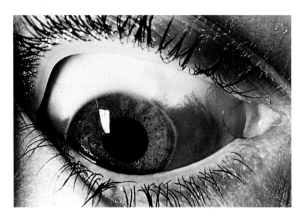

FIGURE 5.10 Subconjunctival hemorrhage. This circumscribed hemorrhage is located between the conjunctiva and the sclera; the history of a sudden appearance and the bright red color are characteristic.

TREATMENT SKILLS

To manage eye injuries properly, every physician should be proficient in ocular irrigation, foreign-body removal, eye medication prescription, and patching.

OCULAR IRRIGATION

Plastic squeeze bottles (Figure 5.11) of eye irrigation solutions and normal saline IV drip with plastic tubing are ideal for ocular irrigation. Irrigation may be facilitated by the use of a topical anesthetic. However, first aid for chemical injuries of the eye may demand the earliest possible irrigation using any source of water available, such as a garden hose, drinking fountain, or faucet. It cannot be overstated that chemical burns require immediate and profuse irrigation. Always direct the irrigating stream toward the temple and away from an unaffected fellow eye.

FOREIGN-BODY REMOVAL

To remove a superficial foreign body from the cornea or conjunctiva, instill a topical anesthetic such as proparacaine 0.5% and then gently roll a cotton-tipped applicator across the globe to pick up the object. A forceful stream of irrigating solution delivered from a squeeze bottle will often dislodge a superficial conjunctival or corneal foreign body. A sharper instrument may be required if the foreign body remains embedded, and the patient should be referred to an ophthalmologist. The

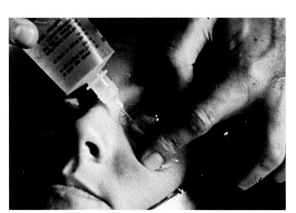

FIGURE 5.11 Irrigation. Here the clinician uses a plastic squeeze bottle of water or normal saline to irrigate the eye. The patient is instructed to look in various directions while the opposite portions of the conjunctival cul-de-sac are flushed vigorously.

orange-brown "rust ring" resulting from an embedded iron foreign body is a common problem that requires special attention.

PRESCRIBING EYE MEDICATION

All physicians should be able to prescribe or administer confidently the following ocular drugs. (See Chapter 9 for more detailed discussions and for the method of administering topical ocular drugs.)

Cycloplegics

Homatropine hydrobromide 5% or cyclopentolate hydrochloride 1% may be used to relax the iris and ciliary body and to relieve the pain and discomfort of most forms of nonpenetrating ocular injuries. Longer-acting cycloplegics (eg, atropine) are usually contraindicated.

Antibiotic Ointment

In general, if employed for 1-time use in clean wounds, antibiotic ointments can be used safely without side effects. If more frequent use is necessary, the possibility of allergic reactions or superinfections must be considered. Gentamicin and neomycin are frequently associated with allergic reaction if used longer than 5 to 7 days.

Anesthetic Eye Drops and Ointment

Ocular anesthetics should never be prescribed for home use because they are toxic to the corneal epithelium when used repeatedly.

PATCHING

Use of a pressure patch or a protective eye shield is indicated in some situations.

Pressure Patch

A moderate pressure patch is used following injuries that affect the corneal epithelium (eg, corneal abrasions) and after removal of foreign bodies. Two eye patches or one eye patch plus a fluffed piece of gauze is applied by putting moderate tension on the strips of tape used (Figure 5.12). Make sure the patch is tight enough to prevent the patient from inadvertently opening the eye under it. The patch should not be so tight as to cause the patient discomfort or severely compress the globe, which can compromise the retinal blood flow.

Shield

For more serious ocular injuries, such as penetration of the globe or hyphema, a shield should be taped over the eye as an interim measure to protect the eye from rubbing, pressure, and further injury prior to treatment by an ophthalmologist. The shield may consist of a perforated, malleable piece of metal (Figure 5.13), plastic, or a trimmed-down paper cup.

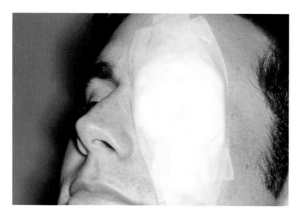

FIGURE 5.12 Pressure patch. The patient is instructed to close both eyes while 1 or more oval, gauze eye patches are taped firmly enough to immobilize the lid of the affected eye in a closed position.

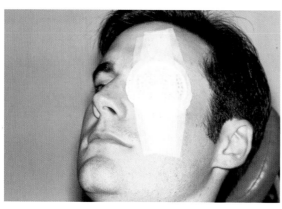

FIGURE 5.13 Shield. Shown here is the Fox shield, made of malleable metal and perforated. The shield is carefully shaped so that the rim of the orbit supports it when taped in place.

SUTURING

The primary care physician can perform suturing of any eyelid skin laceration that does not involve the eyelid margin or the lacrimal canaliculi. More complicated lid lacerations should be referred to an ophthalmologist.

POINTS TO REMEMBER

- Know your limits: do not attempt complex repair, and know the results of inadequate repair.
- Almost without fail, a teardrop-shaped pupil and a flat anterior chamber in an injured eye are associated with a perforating injury of the cornea or of the limbal area. Look for prolapse of dark tissue (either iris or ciliary body) at the point of the teardrop.
- Avoid digital palpation of the globe in any patient who may have a corneal laceration or other perforating injury.
- In a patient with a chemical burn, immediate irrigation is crucial as soon as the nature of the injury has been identified. Do not attempt to neutralize or buffer the chemical substance. The goal is simply to dilute the chemical as thoroughly as possible by copious flushing.
- Traumatic abrasions are generally located in the central or inferior corneal due to the Bell phenomenon (eye rotates superiorly on lid closure). A corneal

abrasion without a history of trauma or an abrasion located in the superior cornea is unusual and may actually represent herpetic epithelial disease, a foreign body under the upper lid, a corneal epithelial dystrophy, or a contact lens–associated disorder.

SAMPLE PROBLEMS

1. Your neighbor, a 43-year-old woman, is cleaning her swimming pool. While she is pouring some concentrated algicide into the pool, a large dollop of this solution splashes into her right eye. You are mowing your lawn when you hear her screams. You come to her aid less than 30 seconds after the injury. Which of the following should you do first?

    a. Bundle her into your car and speed off for the nearest emergency center.
    b. Run back home to get your medical bag where you keep a squeeze bottle of ophthalmic irrigating solution that you can use to flush out her eye.
    c. Run back to your study to look up the specific antidote for algicide.
    d. Carefully examine her eye for evidence of ocular hyperemia.
    e. Dunk her head into the swimming pool, instructing her to hold her eyes open to flush out the chemical.

    Answer: e. This is one of the few true emergencies of all the ocular injuries that you must know. Early and copious irrigation with whatever source of water is handy is the right approach to this problem. Even with prompt treatment, serious ocular injuries and visual damage may result, depending on the offending chemical. Time is of the essence. Do not resort to methods that will cause delay.

2. A 32-year-old man comes to the emergency room with a painful, red eye. He reports that he was riding his bike earlier that morning and felt something hit his eye. He immediately washed the eye with water, but could not relieve the discomfort.

    A. If you suspect that a foreign body is causing the symptoms, what is the best way to exam under the upper lid?

    Answer: The best way to examine for a foreign body under the upper lid is to apply topical anesthetic, evert the lid, and inspect directly.

    B. If he sustained a corneal abrasion and no foreign body is identified, what would you expect on examination?

    a. Increased tearing
    b. Decreased vision
    c. Epithelial defect/staining
    d. Cloudy cornea
    e. Itching

    Answer: a, b, and c. Due to the increased tearing and epithelial defect, the vision is often blurred. A recent corneal abrasion should not be cloudy unless it is an ulcer, which would rarely occur so soon after injury. Itching is a sign of allergic conjunctivitis and is not seen with this diagnosis.

C. Appropriate treatment for a corneal abrasion would be which of the following?

   a. Topical anesthetics to control the pain
   b. Antibiotic eye drops or ointment
   c. Oral antibiotics
   d. Possibly an eye patch to keep lid closed

Answer: b and d. Topical anesthetics should never be prescribed for prolonged use, and oral antibiotics are rarely indicated. The eye may be patched with care to be sure the eyelid remains shut when the other eye is open.

3. If you suspect that a patient has a perforation of the eye, what signs might you expect to see?

   a. Irregular shape to the pupil
   b. Shallow anterior chamber
   c. Low intraocular pressure by digital palpation
   d. Uveal tissue prolapse
   e. Hyphema

Answer: a, b, d, and e. If you suspect a perforation of the eye, digital palpation or any procedure that puts pressure on the eye should not be done.

4. You are on duty in the emergency center when an 18-year-old high school student comes in because of pain, tearing, sensitivity to light, and blurred vision in his right eye. His symptoms began sometime that afternoon. Earlier, he had been working on his car and he remembers something flying into his right eye while he was trying to knock a rivet off the chassis with a hammer and chisel. You examine his eye and take visual acuity measurements. You determine that visual acuity is 20/50 in the right eye and 20/20 in the left eye. There is some conjunctival hyperemia. The pupil of the right eye seems to be peaked and pointing to the 7 o'clock position of the limbus. There is a small, dark, slightly elevated body at the 7 o'clock position of the limbus. You cannot see fundus details of the right eye, but the left eye appears normal. Which of the following would be the appropriate initial management for this situation?

   a. Irrigation of the limbal foreign body
   b. Application of a protective shield
   c. Removal of the limbal foreign body using a cotton-tipped applicator
   d. Removal of the limbal foreign body using forceps
   e. A prescription for topical anesthetic (eg, proparacaine 0.5%) to relieve the patient's symptoms, with strict instructions that he return to see you if his blurred vision continues into the week

Answer: b. Any patient whose recent activities involve striking metal on metal should be suspected of having a foreign body, even with minimal signs and symptoms. However, the case illustrated includes a giveaway sign, namely, peaking of the pupil toward the 7 o'clock position. At that position, the dark body is likely to be iris or ciliary body rather than a foreign body. This indicates a penetrating ocular injury, and the patient should be protected from further eye trauma by a protective shield. A CT scan will confirm the diagnosis of ocular or orbital foreign body. The patient should be referred urgently to an ophthalmologist.

5. While cutting his roses, a neighbor develops a sudden pain in his left eye. Inspection is limited because his eyes are closed, but nothing is visible on external examination.

A. What do you think might have happened?

Answer: Possibilities include a foreign body on the eye or under the lid; a superficial abrasion; or, less likely but still possible, perforation by a thorn.

B. What steps would you need to take to assess and treat this problem?

Answer:

(1) Open the lids gently; never force them open, and never apply pressure to the globe if perforation is suspected. Instill a drop of topical anesthetic, if necessary, to facilitate examination.

(2) Inspect the cornea and the sclera for a foreign body or possible perforation.

(3) Evert the lids to look for a foreign body, unless perforation is suspected.

(4) Remove the foreign body by irrigation or with a cotton-tipped applicator.

(5) Act on any indications for drops, ointment, or patching.

(6) If a possibility of ocular penetration exists, either by examination or history, referral to an ophthalmologist is indicated.

Clinical findings in such cases can be very subtle. Ocular penetration with vegetable matter such as a thorn carries not only the usual risks of ocular penetration (ie, endophthalmitis, cataract, and corneal scar) but also the possibility of a fungal infection.

6. While you are on duty in the emergency center, a patient is brought in who has been involved in a car accident. His face is bloody, especially around the eyes. His history is unclear.

A. What would you do? What would you avoid?

Answer: Cleanse carefully. Avoid pressure of any kind on the eye.

B. While cleansing, you find a cut in the eyelid. It seems easy to stitch, but the lids are swollen and the patient cannot open his eye. What next? Do you stitch the lid?

Answer: First, inspect the eye for possible perforation. Because the lid laceration is not an emergency, stitching is not immediately necessary.

C. If the eye is normal, how should you analyze the problem of the lid laceration?

Answer: The appropriate choice of treatment depends on the level of damage. If only the skin is involved, you may be able to stitch the lid. If the laceration is full-thickness or involves the lid margin, referral to an ophthalmologist is preferred. Any involvement of the canaliculi requires exquisite repair in order to avoid a chronic tearing problem for the rest of the patient's life; referral to an ophthalmologist is mandatory.

7. A 25-year-old man visits the emergency room complaining of decreased vision and pain in his right eye after being involved in a fist fight. Although he has edema and ecchymosis of the eyelids, you are able to examine his eye. His visual acuity is OD 20/70 and OS 20/20, and his pupils are round and reactive. However, the right pupil is sluggish, and shining a light in either eye causes pain in his right eye. He has no restriction of motility. On examination of the anterior segment, you notice a diffuse haze in the anterior chamber and early layering of blood inferiorly. Direct ophthalmoscopy reveals an absent red reflex and no view of the retina is possible. Which of the following would be the most appropriate treatment?

   a. Instill antibiotic ointment and cycloplegic drops, apply a pressure patch, and have the patient follow up with an ophthalmologist in a few days.
   b. Prescribe steroid drops and cycloplegic drops, and tell the patient to keep his head elevated at all times.
   c. Immediately refer the patient to an ophthalmologist to rule out ruptured globe or increased intraocular pressure.

   Answer: c. Although option b may represent appropriate treatment for hyphema, the patient needs to be adequately evaluated for a ruptured globe and peripheral retinal tears. Option a represents treatment for corneal abrasion, not hyphema.

8. An elderly woman falls and hits her face on the coffee table at home. She had some nosebleeding on that side after the fall. She presents to your office 2 hours later with edema and ecchymosis of the eyelids with numbness of the cheek and teeth on that side.

   A. What should be the first priority in the examination?

      a. Palpate the globe to see if the pressure is normal.
      b. Repair any eyelid lacerations.

c. Send the patient for a CT scan to rule out fractures.

d. Carefully open the lids and examine for a ruptured globe.

Answer: d. The first step in any ocular or orbital trauma is to assess the status of the eye and avoid any manipulation of the eye until it is found to be intact.

B. The patient sees 20/20, the pupil is regular, and the eye sustained only a subconjunctival hemorrhage. After appropriate tests, the diagnosis of orbital fracture is made. What would treatment include?

a. Ice packs to the orbit

b. Avoiding blowing the nose

c. Immediate surgical intervention

d. Oral antibiotics

Answer: a, b, and d. Surgical repair of orbital fractures is not an emergency and can be handled over the next 1 to 2 weeks. A referral to an ophthalmologist is indicated in the next few days. Blowing the nose can cause intraorbital emphysema and should be avoided. Ice packs often decrease swelling in an acute event. Because the orbit is now exposed to bacteria in the sinuses, oral antibiotics are warranted.

ANNOTATED RESOURCES

Basic and Clinical Science Course, Section 8: External Disease and Cornea. San Francisco, CA: American Academy of Ophthalmology; updated annually. An excellent summary of anterior segment trauma, covering general principles, burns, superficial injuries, blunt trauma, and perforating injuries.

Kaiser PK, Corneal Abrasion Patching Study Group. A comparison of pressure patching versus no patching for corneal abrasions due to trauma or foreign body removal. *Ophthalmology*. 1995;102:1936–1942. Patients with noninfected non–contact-lens-related traumatic corneal abrasions and abrasions secondary to foreign body removal healed faster with less pain using antibiotics and mydriatics alone, without the need for a pressure patch.

Kaiser PK, Pineda R, Corneal Abrasion Patching Study Group. A study of topical nonsteroidal anti-inflammatory drops and no pressure patching in the treatment of corneal abrasions. *Ophthalmology*. 1997;104:1353–1359. The addition of a topical NSAID to antibiotic treatment of non–contact-lens-related traumatic corneal abrasions increased patient comfort and sped time to resumption of normal activities.

MacCumber MW, ed. *Management of Ocular Injuries and Emergencies*. 4th ed. Philadelphia, PA: Lippincott Williams & Wilkins; 1998. Used widely by ophthalmology residents, this book contains extensive information useful to the student or emergency center physician who desires more information on serious eye trauma.

Newell FW. *Ophthalmology: Principles and Concepts*. 8th ed. St Louis, MO: CV Mosby; 1996. Ocular injuries are summarized succinctly in "Injuries of the Eye" in this comprehensive textbook.

Trobe JD. *The Physician's Guide to Eye Care*. 3rd ed. San Francisco, CA: American Academy of Ophthalmology; 2006. A brief but comprehensive resource covering the principal clinical ophthalmic problems that nonophthalmologist physicians are likely to encounter, organized for practical use by practitioners.

Amblyopia and Strabismus

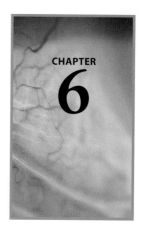

OBJECTIVES

As a primary care physician, you should be able to recognize the signs and symptoms of amblyopia and strabismus; be able to perform the necessary tests to screen for these conditions; and, if the patient is a child, be cognizant of the need to arrange for prompt ophthalmologic consultation, particularly when intraocular disease is suspected. To achieve these objectives, you should learn to

> ➤ Measure or estimate visual acuity in children
> ➤ Detect strabismus by general inspection, the corneal light reflex test, and the cover test
> ➤ Perform ophthalmoscopy in a child to rule out any organic causes of impaired vision when amblyopia is suspected
> ➤ Explain to parents the need for prompt treatment of amblyopia

RELEVANCE

Amblyopia is a form of treatable visual loss found in approximately 2% of the young adult population of the United States. It can be defined as a loss of visual acuity not correctable by glasses in an otherwise healthy eye. Amblyopia develops in infancy or early childhood and usually can be detected in very young patients, principally by measuring or estimating visual acuity. If detected and treated early, amblyopia can be cured. For best results, treatment should begin before age 5; treatment for amblyopia is rarely successful if initiated past age 10. If amblyopia is not detected and treated early in life, visual impairment from amblyopia persists for the patient's entire lifetime. At least half of all patients with amblyopia also have strabismus, a misalignment of the 2 eyes.

The pediatrician or family physician will most likely be the first to see a young patient with amblyopia or strabismus and, therefore, will have the principal responsibility for screening. The child's physician must be familiar with the different kinds of amblyopia and strabismus, the close relationship of these 2 conditions, and how best to detect them.

BASIC INFORMATION

Vision is a developmental sensory function. Vision at birth is relatively poor, but through proper visual stimulation in the early months and years of life, a normal acuity is achieved at about 3 years of age. If this developmental process—the stimulation of the vision-receptive cells in the brain—is prevented because of strabismus, abnormal refractive error, congenital cataract, or some other condition, vision will not develop properly. This is a failure of the developmental process, not primarily an organic abnormality of the eye.

AMBLYOPIA

Amblyopia is a reduction in visual acuity in the absence of detectable organic disease (such as cataract, retinoblastoma, or other inflammatory or congenital ocular disorders) that results from a disruption of the normal development of vision. It is usually unilateral, but it can (rarely) affect both eyes. Amblyopia does not cause learning disorders.

Amblyopia may develop in young children who receive visual information from one eye that is blurred or conflicts with information from the other eye. To understand how amblyopia may develop in this way, consider that the brain is receiving 2 stimuli for each visual event: 1 from a visually aligned (fixating) eye and 1 from an "abnormal" eye (vision blurred or eye misaligned). If this abnormal visual experience is prolonged, the brain continually "favors" the eye with better vision, to the eventual detriment of visual development in the other eye. For this reason, amblyopia is often referred to colloquially as "lazy eye."

A number of predisposing factors can lead to the development of amblyopia. These are summarized below.

Strabismic Amblyopia

A child can develop amblyopia in the context of strabismus (misaligned eyes, Figure 6.1). The eye used habitually for fixation retains normal acuity and the nonpreferred eye often develops decreased vision. Adult-onset strabismus generally will cause diplopia (double vision) because the 2 eyes are not aligned on the same object. The brain of a child, on the other hand, is more adaptive. In a similar strabismic situation, the child's brain ignores (suppresses) the image from one of the eyes—usually the one that provides the blurrier image.

Sometimes the degree of misalignment between the 2 eyes is very slight, making detection of strabismus and suspicion of strabismic amblyopia difficult. Even with a small angle of strabismus, amblyopia may be quite severe.

Refractive Amblyopia

Amblyopia can result from a difference in refractive error between the 2 eyes. The eye with the lesser refractive error provides the clearer image and usually is favored over the other eye; consequently, amblyopia develops. Children with asymmetric hyperopia are susceptible, because unequal accommodation is impossible; the child

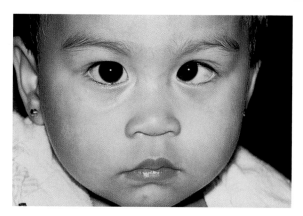

FIGURE 6.1 Strabismus. Strabismus is the most common underlying cause of amblyopia. With constant deviation of 1 eye, reduced vision occurs. Amblyopia is less likely when the deviation is intermittent or when the 2 eyes alternate fixation. (Reprinted from "Understanding and Preventing Amblyopia." In: *Eye Care Skills: Presentations for Physicians and Other Health Care Professionals,* v3.0. San Francisco, CA: American Academy of Ophthalmology; 2009.)

can bring only 1 eye at a time into focus. Refractive amblyopia may be as severe as that found in strabismic amblyopia. However, the pediatrician or family physician may overlook the possibility of amblyopia because there is no obvious strabismus. Detection of amblyopia must be based on an abnormality found in visual acuity testing.

Form-Deprivation and Occlusion Amblyopia

Form-deprivation amblyopia (amblyopia ex anopsia) can result when opacities of the ocular media—such as cataracts (Figure 6.2), corneal scarring, or even drooping of the upper lid (ptosis)—prevent adequate sensory input and thus disrupt visual development. The amblyopia can persist even when the cause of the media

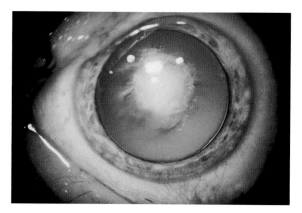

FIGURE 6.2 Opacities of the ocular media. Congenital cataract, if significant, should be removed within the first few months of life. Good vision can be obtained if the cataract is removed and the refractive error corrected. (Reprinted from "Understanding and Preventing Amblyopia." In: *Eye Care Skills: Presentations for Physicians and Other Health Care Professionals,* v3.0. San Francisco, CA: American Academy of Ophthalmology; 2009.)

opacity or ptosis is corrected. Rarely, occlusion amblyopia can result from patching of the normal eye.

STRABISMUS

Strabismus is a misalignment of the 2 eyes, so that both eyes cannot be directed toward the object of regard. Strabismus may cause or be caused by the absence of binocular vision; as with amblyopia, strabismus does not cause learning disabilities.

It is clinically useful to distinguish between concomitant (nonparalytic) and incomitant (paralytic or restrictive) strabismus. Additionally, a number of terms are used to describe and classify strabismus. These distinctions and terms are summarized below.

Concomitant Strabismus

Strabismus is called *concomitant* or *nonparalytic* when the angle (or degree) of misalignment is approximately equal in all directions of gaze (Figure 6.3). The individual extraocular muscles are functioning normally, but the 2 eyes are simply not directed toward the same target. Most concomitant strabismus has its onset in childhood. In children, it often causes the secondary development of suppression to overcome double vision and thus leads to strabismic amblyopia. Concomitant strabismus in patients under age 6 is rarely caused by serious neurologic disease. Strabismus arising later in life may have a specific and serious neurologic basis. Concomitant strabismus may occur in an adult who loses most or all of the vision in one eye from intraocular or optic nerve disease. A blind eye in an adult will frequently drift outward, while in a child the eye will turn inward.

Incomitant Strabismus

Strabismus is called *incomitant*, *paralytic*, or *restrictive* when the degree of misalignment varies with the direction of gaze (Figure 6.4). One or more of the extraocular muscles or nerves may not be functioning properly, or normal movement may be mechanically restricted. This type of strabismus may well indicate either a serious neurologic disorder, such as third cranial nerve paresis (see Chapter 7), or orbital

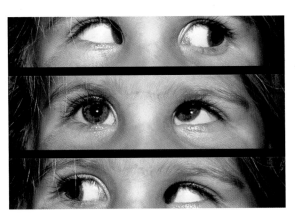

FIGURE 6.3 Concomitant strabismus. In the views presented here, the misaligned eyes exhibit about the same degree of inward deviation (esotropia) in each position of gaze.

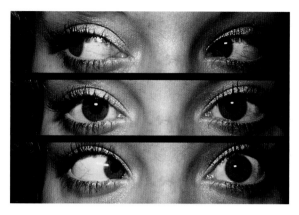

FIGURE 6.4 Incomitant strabismus. The eyes appear straight in right gaze (top) and straight-ahead gaze (middle), but a misalignment is obvious in left gaze (bottom), indicating a paralysis of the left lateral rectus muscle or a restriction of the left medial rectus. These eye positions would be found in a left sixth cranial nerve palsy.

disease or trauma, such as the restrictive ophthalmopathy of thyroid disease or a blowout fracture.

Heterophoria and Heterotropia

Heterophoria is a latent tendency for misalignment of the 2 eyes that becomes manifest only if binocular vision is interrupted, such as by covering 1 eye. During binocular viewing, the 2 eyes of a patient with heterophoria are aligned perfectly; both eyes are directed at the same object of regard. However, when 1 eye is covered, that eye will drift to its position of rest. Once the cover is removed, the eye will realign itself with the other eye. A minor degree of heterophoria is normal for most individuals.

Heterotropia is really another term for strabismus. In general, *tropia* refers to a manifest deviation that is present when both eyes are open (no covers). Usually, binocular vision is reduced. Some patients, however, can demonstrate an intermittent heterotropia and thus achieve binocular vision part of the time.

Heterotropia and heterophoria can be subdivided further according to the direction of the deviation involved. In esotropia and esophoria, the deviating eye is directed inward toward the nose. Esotropia is a manifest deviation and is the most common type of deviation in childhood. Exotropia is much more likely to be intermittent than esotropia, with an outward deviation of an eye alternating with alignment of the eyes. Children with this condition suppress double vision when the deviating eye is turned out and achieve some degree of binocular vision when the 2 eyes are straight. Vertical heterotropias and heterophorias have many different causes, including paralysis or dysfunction of vertically acting extraocular muscles. When vertical deviations are described, the deviating eye (right or left) should be specified. Table 6.1 summarizes the directions of deviation in heterophoria and heterotropia. Figure 6.5 depicts the different kinds of heterotropia.

HOW TO EXAMINE AND INTERPRET THE FINDINGS

Pediatric vision screening is important for detecting not only amblyopia and strabismus but also congenital cataract, glaucoma, retinoblastoma, and other

TABLE 6.1 Summary of Heterophoria and Heterotropia

PREFIX	NAME OF DISORDER		DESCRIPTION
	-phoria (latent)	-tropia (manifest)	
eso-	esophoria	esotropia	inward deviation
exo-	exophoria	exotropia	outward deviation
hyper-	hyperphoria	hypertropia	upward deviation
hypo-	hypophoria	hypotropia	downward deviation

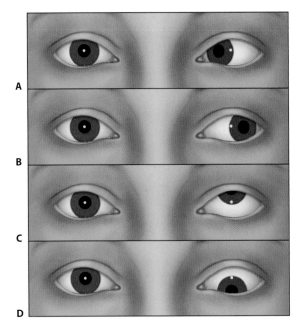

FIGURE 6.5 Types of heterotropia. Note the corneal light reflex. **A.** Esotropia (inward). **B.** Exotropia (outward). **C.** Hypertropia (upward). **D.** Hypotropia (downward). (Illustration by Christine Gralapp, MA, CMI)

vision-threatening or life-threatening conditions. Regular screening by the pediatrician or family physician helps ensure that the child's vision is developing normally or, if it is not, that early treatment is instituted. At a minimum, all children should undergo an evaluation to detect eye and vision abnormalities during the first few months of life and again at about age 3.

Visual acuity testing is important for detecting amblyopia as well as refractive error, which can lead to amblyopia in young children. Strabismus may be detected by general inspection, the corneal light reflex test, or the cover test. Additional tests are important for general eye screening in children of all ages: pupillary reactions are important in assessing normal eye function and health; direct ophthalmoscopy is required to detect media opacities by eliciting a red reflex and to examine the fundus for retinal abnormalities. These techniques are discussed later in the chapter.

AMBLYOPIA TESTING

Amblyopia can be detected by testing the visual acuity in each eye separately. Although there is no specific Mendelian pattern of inheritance, strabismus and amblyopia sometimes cluster in families. Restoration of normal visual acuity can be successful only if treatment is instituted during the first decade of life, when the visual system is still in the formative stage. Techniques for measuring or estimating visual acuity (or visual function) and detecting amblyopia vary with the child's age, as described below.

Newborns

True visual acuity is difficult to measure in newborns. However, infants' general ocular status should be assessed through corneal light reflex testing, evaluation of the red reflex, pupillary testing, and, if possible, fundus examination.

Infants to 2-Year-Olds

With infants, it is possible only to assess visual function, not visual acuity. To test for amblyopia in infants (from a few months to about age 2), cover each eye in turn with the hand or, preferably, an adhesive patch and note how the child reacts. The infant should be able to maintain central fixation with each eye. If amblyopia is present, the child will likely protest—vocally or by evasive movements—the covering of the "good" eye. Visual function, including ocular motility, may be further assessed by passing an interesting object, such as a ring of keys, before the baby and noting how the infant watches and follows the moving object. Moving the child's head can be used to demonstrate full ocular motility if not otherwise documented by following movements.

Age 2 to 4 or 5

A picture card (Figure 6.6) may be used to test visual acuity in children between 2 and 3 years of age. At age 3 (or before, if the child can follow directions and communicate adequately), visual acuity can be tested with the tumbling E chart (Figure 6.7). In the tumbling E test, the child is asked to point with his or her fingers to indicate the direction of the "arms" of the E. The HOTV test is another vision assessment for preliterate children (Figure 6.8). A card with the 4 very distinct letters H, O, T, and V, is given to the child. One of the letters is highlighted on the chart, and the child points to the appropriate letter. Use of an adhesive patch is the best way to ensure full monocular occlusion and accurate acuity measurement in children at these ages (Figure 6.9).

Vision should be rechecked annually once visual acuity has been determined to be normal in each eye. Young children may not quite reach 20/20 acuity; this is no cause for concern as long as vision is at least 20/40 and both eyes are equal. A recent advance in early detection of amblyogenic factors is photoscreening. A computerized camera takes photographs of the child's undilated eyes. Refractive errors, strabismus, anisometropia, and media opacities are visible in the photos. This

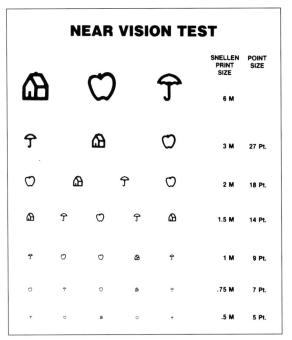

NEAR VISION TEST

FIGURE 6.6 Picture card. This figure shows one type of picture card used to test visual acuity in young children. To use the picture card, the examiner familiarizes the child with the pictures at close range. Each eye is then tested individually at a testing distance of 6 meters (20 feet) from the child by asking the child to name the various objects.

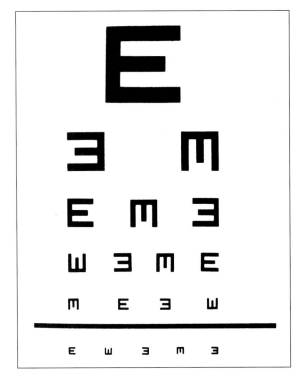

FIGURE 6.7 Tumbling E chart. Visual acuity testing in children should be done at 6 meters (20 feet) with charts such as the tumbling E shown here. The child indicates the direction of the "arms" of the E by pointing with their fingers.

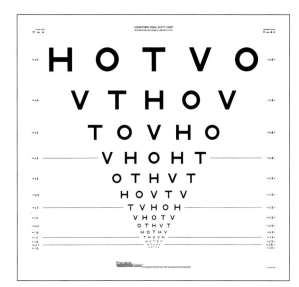

FIGURE 6.8 HOTV chart. The child is given a handheld chart with the letters HOTV on it and is asked to point to the letter that is highlighted on an eyechart with the same letters, HOTV, on it. (Reprinted from Hartmann EE, et al. Preschool vision screening: summary of a task force report. *Ophthalmology.* 2001;108:482.)

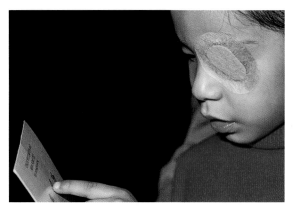

FIGURE 6.9 Measuring visual acuity. This becomes possible by age 2 to 4 years. An adhesive patch to cover the eye not being tested helps to facilitate the exam as well as to prevent "peeking." (Reprinted from "Understanding and Preventing Amblyopia. A Slide-Script Program." San Francisco, CA: American Academy of Ophthalmology; 1987:12.)

technique permits screening of preverbal children and those unable to cooperate with other types of testing. Photoscreening is not a substitute for accurate visual acuity measurement, but it can provide significant information about factors that may lead to amblyopia.

Age 4 or 5 and Up

The Snellen chart may be used to test visual acuity in children age 4 or 5 and up who know the letters of the alphabet (see Chapter 1).

STRABISMUS TESTING

Strabismus testing for children (and adults) consists of general inspection, the corneal light reflex test, and the cover test. These techniques are described below.

Children up to age 3 or 4 months may exhibit temporary uncoordinated eye movements and intermittent strabismus. However, if occasional deviation persists beyond this age, a referral to an ophthalmologist should be made. Constant deviations should be referred at any age.

Epicanthus (Figure 6.10), in which epicanthal skin folds extend toward the upper eyelid and brow and the nose bridge is flat, may give an infant the appearance of esotropia, especially if the head or eyes are turned slightly to the right or left. As the child's head grows and the nose bridge develops, the epicanthus becomes less obvious. This may be mistakenly interpreted as the child outgrowing presumed strabismus; however, a child does not outgrow a true strabismus. The cover test and evaluation of the corneal light reflex will distinguish between pseudostrabismus (epicanthus) and true strabismus. However, it is important to keep in mind that strabismus can also occur in the presence of epicanthus.

General Inspection

For infants and older children, a general inspection may reveal an identifiable deviation of one eye. Having the patient look in the 6 cardinal positions of gaze (Figure 6.11) may reveal whether the deviation is approximately the same in all fields—indicating concomitant strabismus—or is significantly different in 1 field of gaze—indicating a possible incomitant strabismus. Involuntary eye jerks known as *nystagmus* may be detected in primary or other fields of gaze. The patient may assume an abnormal head posture (ie, a tilt or turn to one side) to reduce the nystagmus and improve the visual acuity or to obtain binocular vision in cases of congenital cranial-nerve palsy. All infants or children with nystagmus should be examined and followed up by an ophthalmologist.

Corneal Light Reflex

Observation of the corneal light reflex constitutes an objective assessment of ocular alignment. Certainly in newborns and often in young children, it may be the only feasible method of testing for strabismus.

The patient is directed to look at a penlight held directly in front of the eyes by the examiner at a distance of 2 feet. The examiner aligns his or her eye with the light source and compares the position of the light as reflected by the cornea of each eye (Figure 6.12). Normally, the light is reflected on each cornea symmetrically and in the same position relative to the pupil and visual axis of each eye. In a deviating eye, the light reflection will be eccentrically positioned and in a direction opposite

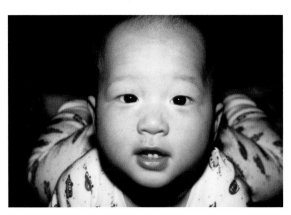

FIGURE 6.10 Epicanthus. An extended lid fold and a relatively flat nose bridge may give the false appearance of an esotropia. (Courtesy Robert T. Lee, MD)

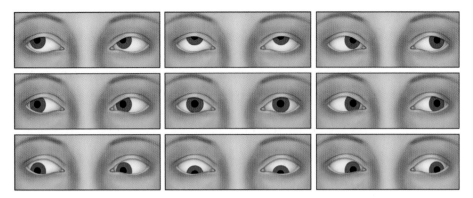

FIGURE 6.11 Positions of gaze. Eye movement can be evaluated by directing the patient to turn the eyes in 6 cardinal positions of gaze: up/right, right, down/right, down/left, left, and up/left. Also shown are the upward gaze, primary gaze, and downward gaze (middle column). (Illustration by Christine Gralapp, MA, CMI)

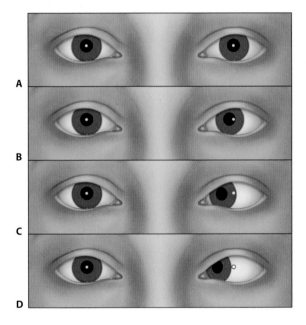

FIGURE 6.12 Corneal light reflex. The position of the light reflection indicates (**A**) a normal alignment, (**B**) a small esotropia, (**C**) a moderate esotropia, and (**D**) a large left esotropia. (Illustration by Christine Gralapp, MA, CMI)

to that of the deviation. The size of the deviation can be estimated by the amount of displacement of the light reflex, but this is a relatively gross estimate.

Cover Test

The cover test (Figure 6.13) is easy to perform, requires no special equipment, and detects almost every case of tropia. It can be used on any patient over the age of 6 or 7 months. To perform the test, have the patient look at a fixation point, such as a detailed or interesting target (eg, a toy) or the Snellen chart. Note which eye seems to be the fixating eye. Cover the fixating eye and observe the other eye. If the uncovered eye moves to pick up the fixation, then it can be reasoned that this eye was not directed toward the object of regard originally (ie, when both eyes

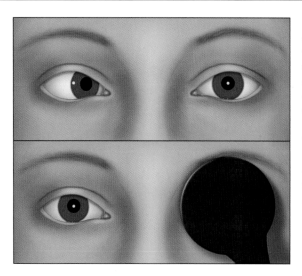

FIGURE 6.13 Cover test. The cover test can be used to screen for strabismus. The results depicted here indicate a right esotropia. When the left eye is covered, the right eye moves outward to pick up fixation. (When the left eye is uncovered, the left eye moves outward to pick up fixation and both eyes assume their original positions.) (Illustration by Christine Gralapp, MA, CMI)

were uncovered). If the eye moves inward to fixate, then originally it must have been deviated outward and hence is exotropic. If the eye moves outward to fixate, then it was deviated inward and is esotropic. If the eye moves up or down, then it is hypotropic or hypertropic, respectively; the deviating eye must be specified in a hypertropia or hypotropia. Of course, each eye must be tested separately because there is no way of knowing which eye may be expressing the deviation.

No shift on cover testing means there is no tropia, but a phoria could still be present. A phoria is detected by alternate cover testing. Each eye is alternately occluded, and the examiner observes the uncovered eye for a refixation shift. The patient has an esophoria if the uncovered eye moves outward to fixate and an exophoria if the eye moves inward to fixate.

A very small-angle deviation may be difficult to detect by evaluating the corneal light reflex or performing the cover test. For this reason, visual acuity testing is important in all cases of suspected strabismus for detection of amblyopia.

OTHER TESTS

The following tests are part of general screening for all children.

Pupillary Testing

Abnormal pupillary responses may indicate neurologic disease or other ocular defects. (Pupillary testing is discussed in Chapter 1; for further discussion and specific techniques see Chapter 7.)

Red Reflex

Light is reflected off the fundus as red when it is examined through the ophthalmoscope from a distance of about 1 foot (Figure 6.14). Media opacities appear in the red reflex as black silhouettes. Leukocoria ("white pupil") is a white reflex that may signify the presence of cataract or retinoblastoma (Figure 6.15).

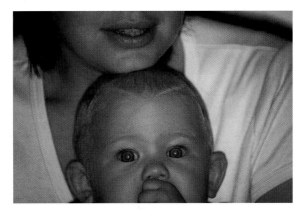

FIGURE 6.14 Evaluation of amblyopia. Assessing the red reflex allows the examiner to evaluate for 2 potential causes of amblyopia: media opacities and high refractive errors. The cornea, anterior chamber, lens, and vitreous must all be clear to allow a view of the retina. If the eye is unusually hyperopic or myopic, the red reflex may be very dim unless the ophthalmoscope's high-power lenses are used. (Modified from "Understanding and Preventing Amblyopia." In: *Eye Care Skills: Presentations for Physicians and Other Health Care Professionals,* v3.0. San Francisco, CA: American Academy of Ophthalmology; 2009.)

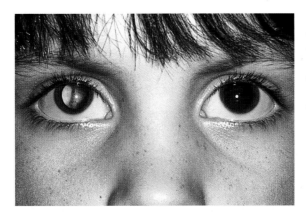

FIGURE 6.15 Leukocoria. A cataract is not the only cause of a white reflex. In this child, a retinoblastoma fills the vitreous cavity. Any change from the normal red reflex warrants careful ophthalmic examination.

All infants and children should be evaluated for the red reflex; pupillary dilation may be necessary to achieve a red reflex (phenylephrine 1.0% and cyclopentolate 0.2% in infants, readily available in combination as Cyclomydril). Other alternatives are 2.5% phenylephrine and 0.5% cyclopentolate in the more deeply pigmented infant. (Caution: cyclopentolate can cause paralytic ileus in premature and neonatal infants.) If the examiner cannot elicit a red reflex, the infant or child should be referred to an ophthalmologist urgently.

Ophthalmoscopy

A careful ophthalmoscopic examination of both eyes through dilated pupils is mandatory for any patient with reduced vision or with strabismus. In this way, the examiner can detect potentially serious intraocular lesions, such as cataract, malignancies such as retinoblastoma, or other abnormalities.

MANAGEMENT OR REFERRAL

The early detection of amblyopia and strabismus is an important responsibility for those involved in infant and child health care. Delayed diagnosis may have serious consequences for visual acuity, eye disease, or systemic disease. If an abnormality is suspected, the patient should be referred promptly to an ophthalmologist.

AMBLYOPIA

In children younger than 5, strabismic amblyopia can usually be treated effectively by the ophthalmologist through occlusion of the unaffected eye (Figure 6.16). The child wears an adhesive patch over the good eye, forcing the brain to utilize the previously nonpreferred eye. In general, the success of occlusion treatment for amblyopia patients between the ages of 5 and 9 will depend on the age of the patient, the degree of the amblyopia, and the persistence of patient compliance with treatment. Treatment is better tolerated by younger children but can be successful in children as old as 18. A treatment program started early in life often must be continued throughout the patient's first decade. Amblyopia treatment by patch occlusion of the unaffected eye must be monitored carefully, especially during the younger years, to avoid causing amblyopia through sensory deprivation of the occluded eye. New studies show that over a quarter of older children with moderate amblyopia will also respond to amblyopic therapy.

Treatment of refractive amblyopia consists first of wearing glasses, followed by patching of the better eye if the visual acuity difference persists after 4 to 8 weeks of wear. Equal vision in both eyes is readily achievable with parental cooperation in almost all cases. In general, the earlier the individual with amblyopia is diagnosed and treated, the better the chance of achieving equal vision. An alternative to occlusion therapy with an adhesive patch is the use of dilating drops (atropine 1%) daily to the better-seeing eye. This blurs the vision in the better-seeing eye and forces the child to use the amblyopic eye.

After cessation of treatment, the child must be monitored for recurrence of amblyopia. This most commonly occurs in the first 3 months after discontinuation of amblyopia therapy.

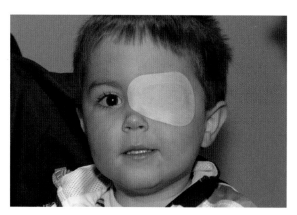

FIGURE 6.16 Reversing amblyopia. Patching (occlusion) of the eye with better vision may be prescribed to help reverse amblyopia. Compliance and follow-up are important. (Courtesy R. Michael Siatkowski, MD)

STRABISMUS

The most effective way to support fusion (binocular vision) is to treat the amblyopia and equalize the vision. Glasses can treat some or all of the esotropia in a farsighted, or hyperopic, individual (Figure 6.17) and may decrease the frequency of deviation in a myopic individual with exotropia. However, surgical correction of the misalignment may still be necessary, particularly in those children who develop esotropia before the age of 6 months (congenital esotropia). Even when binocular vision may not be achievable, the impact of a disfiguring strabismus on a patient's self-image is a valid indication for surgery. It must be stressed that surgery is not an alternative to glasses and patching when amblyopia is present. "Vision training" has no proven value for the treatment of amblyopia or strabismus.

SERIOUS INTRAOCULAR LESIONS

Ocular abnormalities such as leukocoria or glaucoma require immediate referral to an ophthalmologist. Leukocoria may be the presenting sign for intraocular tumors such as retinoblastoma or for a visually significant cataract. Both conditions require prompt ophthalmic treatment. Glaucoma presents in the infant with photophobia and tearing, corneal enlargement, and clouding (Figure 6.18). If glaucoma is suspected, immediate referral to an ophthalmologist is indicated.

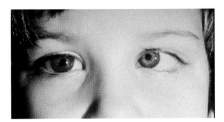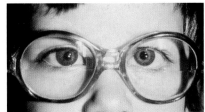

FIGURE 6.17 Esotropia. An inward turning of the eye, esotropia is the most common type of strabismus. About one-half of all cases of strabismus are due to a form of esotropia caused by excessive focusing, or accommodation. Accommodative esotropia frequently begins as an intermittent crossing and gradually becomes constant. The age of onset is usually about 2 years, but may be as late as 7. This child is farsighted and, without glasses, accommodates to see, resulting in crossed eyes. Glasses relieve this accommodative demand, enabling the eyes to straighten.

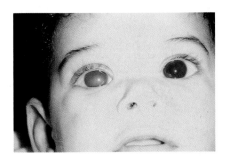

FIGURE 6.18 Glaucoma. Enlarged, cloudy cornea in a child with congenital glaucoma. (Reprinted from *Basic and Clinical Science Course*, Section 6: Pediatric Ophthalmology and Strabismus. San Francisco, CA: American Academy of Ophthalmology; 2009–2010:273.)

POINTS TO REMEMBER

- Amblyopia must be detected early and referred to an ophthalmologist to be treated successfully.
- The importance of visual acuity testing in detecting amblyopia cannot be overemphasized. Amblyopia may be present in eyes without strabismus, so the vision in each eye may not be normal even if the eyes appear normally aligned.
- Several serious organic conditions cause strabismus as one manifestation of the disease; therefore, all patients with strabismus should be referred to an ophthalmologist at the time of diagnosis for further testing.
- Children may have cataracts, glaucoma, and retinal diseases, so children with unusually large eye(s), decreased or no red reflex, or poor vision should be referred to an ophthalmologist.
- Vision training has no proven value in the treatment of amblyopia or strabismus.

SAMPLE PROBLEMS

1. A 3-year-old girl is brought to you by her father, who tells you that he suspects his daughter's right eye is not straight. What steps would you take to determine if a significant problem is present?

   Answer: First, visual acuity testing should be attempted using the tumbling E chart or a picture card, with each eye alternately covered by an adhesive patch. A difference in visual acuity between the eyes or decreased vision in both eyes is significant. Then test the alignment of the eyes by evaluating the corneal light reflex and performing the cover test. Unequal positioning of the light reflex or movement of the uncovered eye to pick up the fixation would suggest a misalignment of the eyes. Next, perform an ophthalmoscopic examination, preferably through dilated pupils, to determine if there is any intraocular basis for visual loss, such as cataract, retinoblastoma, or a retinal abnormality. If there is a suspicion of intraocular disease, the patient should be referred for an urgent ophthalmologic evaluation. If visual acuity is reduced in one or both eyes, or if misalignment of the eyes is detected, a nonurgent referral should be made.

2. A family has just moved into your area and the mother brings her 6-month-old baby to your family practice office for a routine checkup. She mentions that the child's grandfather has noted that in several photographs the baby's left eye appears crossed. He is adamant in his observation and feels that "something should be done." The mother has felt that, at times, the eye has appeared crossed, but the baby's father has not observed this phenomenon. How should you proceed?

   Answer: Inquire about any family history of strabismus or amblyopia and evaluate for the presence of epicanthus. Place your hand in front of one eye and then the other to see if the child exhibits displeasure. Observe the alignment of the child's eyes as well as extraocular movements if possible. Use a penlight to assess the position of the corneal light reflex. The direct ophthalmoscope can be used to evaluate the red reflex and the fundus. Examination reveals that significant epicanthal lid folds are present. The corneal light reflex is the same in each eye, and full extraocular movements are seen in all cardinal positions of gaze. Although in this case the appearance of a crossed eye is probably the result of epicanthus, continued observation on the next visit is indicated. Remember that strabismus and amblyopia can occur in a patient with epicanthus, and the strabismus may be intermittent. Any suspected abnormality should be referred to an ophthalmologist.

3. A 2-year-old boy is brought to your office because his mother has noticed that over the past 2 weeks his right eye has deviated inward during periods of fatigue. On the previous evening, the boy's father claimed to have noted a white reflex in the child's right eye. How should you proceed?

    Answer: Show the child a toy and cover his left eye with your hand; evaluate his response. Cover his right eye to compare his response. Evaluate the corneal light reflex and perform the cover test. In particular, note whether an abnormal response is elicited on covering one eye. Test the pupillary light reflexes. Perform an ophthalmoscopic examination, preferably through a dilated pupil, to assess the red reflex and observe for organic pathology.

    Examination reveals equal pupillary light reflexes. The red reflex appears white (leukocoria) on ophthalmoscopic examination of the right eye as compared with the left. No detail can be seen in the right fundus. Your findings indicate the need for an urgent referral. Ophthalmologic consultation determined that the esotropia in this child occurred secondary to a retinoblastoma.

4. A 54-year-old woman has early cataracts in both eyes. With glasses, the right eye cannot be corrected to better than 20/200, whereas with the left eye she can read the 20/40 line with best correction. The amount of cataract is exactly the same in each eye. Examination of the optic disc and macula, pupillary reaction, color vision, and retinal blood vessels proved entirely normal in each eye. However, the right eye appears to be turned slightly inward when you evaluate the corneal light reflex, and the patient has not experienced diplopia. Additional questioning reveals that the patient wore a patch over one eye as a child. Why would information concerning her childhood ocular condition be relevant in this situation?

    Answer: The poor vision in the right eye may be due to long-standing amblyopia. If this is the case, an ophthalmologist will conclude that removal of the cataract would result in vision only as good as that during the adolescent years. This information is valuable in helping to determine if cataract surgery on the right eye is likely to be helpful to the patient.

5. A 4-year-old boy with attention-deficit disorder comes to your office for his routine preschool physical examination. Your nurse tests his visual acuity with the picture card and obtains 20/30 vision on the right. During testing of the left eye the patient loses attention and refuses to cooperate further with testing. What course of action should you take?

   Answer: Often children become uncooperative with visual acuity testing due to poor vision in the eye being tested. This is sometimes misinterpreted as a behavioral rather than an ocular issue. This patient can return on another day to have the left eye tested first, with the right eye covered by an adhesive patch. If visual acuity measurement is still unsuccessful, the patient should be referred to an ophthalmologist for evaluation.

6. A 4-year-old girl is brought to your office by her mother, who says that she sees her daughter's right eye "drifting." You test the patient's vision, which is 20/20 in each eye. There is no epicanthus. The corneal light test shows no deviation, and the cover test fails to reveal strabismus. What is your next step?

   Answer: Strabismus can be intermittent. Intermittent esodeviations are usually early manifestations of a constant deviation and may be difficult to detect during the early stages. Intermittent exodeviations are more pronounced when the patient is tired or sick but can be easily missed. If the patient has a reliable history of strabismus but you are unable to detect the deviation, referral to an ophthalmologist is recommended.

7. A mother reports that her 1-year-old child is sensitive to light, and his right eye looks larger than the left. On examination, you note that although the child's right eye does look larger, the pupillary reactions are equal in both eyes, the corneas are clear, and there is a good red reflex in each eye. What should you tell the mother?

   a. Do not worry, the child will "grow into" his eyes.
   b. Return in 1 month for a reexamination.
   c. Take the child to an ophthalmologist on my referral.
   d. This is probably a cancer of the right eye, and you should take the child to an oncologist on my referral.

   Answer: c. Children can have glaucoma, which causes buphthalmos, or enlargement of one or both eyes. Although glaucoma may be associated with increased tearing, sensitivity to light, and a hazy or white cornea, the only sign of glaucoma in some children may be enlargement of the eye or eyes. This child should be referred immediately to an ophthalmologist for diagnosis and management.

8. A 60-year-old man comes to see you because of the sudden onset of double vision. He states that when he looks straight ahead, he does not have diplopia,

but on right gaze he has diplopia, with the 2 images horizontally displaced. He has no other abnormal neurologic symptoms. His past medical history is significant for diabetes mellitus. How would you assess this patient?

Answer: First, check the visual acuity in each eye and test the pupillary light reflexes. Observe the corneal light reflex, and perform a cover test. It is important to observe the patient's eye movements in all the cardinal positions of gaze. He may have an incomitant strabismus that can be seen in only some fields of gaze. If an incomitant strabismus is detected, he may have a cranial nerve palsy. Ophthalmologic and neurologic consultation should be obtained emergently.

ANNOTATED RESOURCES

Johns KJ, ed. Understanding and preventing amblyopia. In: *Eye Care Skills: Presentations for Physicians and Other Health Care Professionals*. San Fancisco, CA: American Academy of Ophthalmology; 2009.

Pediatric Eye Disease Investigator Group. A randomized trial of atropine vs. patching for treatment of moderate amblyopia in children. *Arch Ophthalmol.* 2002;120:268–278.

Pediatric Eye Disease Investigator Group. Randomized trial of treatment of amblyopia in children age 7 to 17 years. *Arch Ophthalmol.* 2005;123: 437–447.

Trobe JD. *The Physician's Guide to Eye Care*. 3rd ed. San Francisco, CA: American Academy of Ophthalmology; 2006. A brief but comprehensive resource covering the principal clinical ophthalmic problems that nonophthalmologist physicians are likely to encounter, organized for practical use by practitioners.

Vaughan DG, Asbury T, Riordan-Eva P. *General Ophthalmology*. 17th ed. Norwalk, CT: Appleton & Lange; 2007. The chapter on strabismus is a well-illustrated, comprehensive review of the subject.

Wright KW. *Pediatric Ophthalmology for Primary Care*. 3rd ed. Elk Grove Village, IL: American Academy of Pediatrics; 2007. The chapter on amblyopia and strabismus is an excellent overview, with great clinical photographs.

Neuro-Ophthalmology

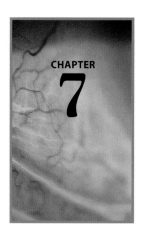

OBJECTIVES

Neuro-ophthalmology is a subspecialty of both neurology and ophthalmology that investigates visual disturbances resulting from disorders of the central nervous system. As a primary care physician, you should learn to

➤ Recognize the signs and symptoms of key neuro-ophthalmic disorders

➤ Obtain a focused neuro-ophthalmic history and examination

➤ Provide a differential diagnosis so that appropriate workup, treatment, and/or consultations may be obtained

RELEVANCE

The visual and oculomotor pathways reflect the status of much of the central nervous system. It is estimated that 40% of the brain is involved with vision, visual processing, eye movement, and ocular stabilization. As a result, many important diseases of the central nervous system can exhibit visual symptoms. An understanding of neuro-ophthalmologic examination techniques and disorders allow the primary care physician to identify potentially life-threatening or vision-threatening neurologic disorders such as brain tumors, multiple sclerosis, cerebrovascular disease, giant cell arteritis, and intracranial aneurysms.

HOW TO EXAMINE

Although the ocular examination is covered in depth in Chapter 1, what follows is a brief review of the eye examination focusing on components essential to neuro-ophthalmology. The neuro-ophthalmologic examination may be simplified to the point where only a few minutes of the physician's time are required, or detailed enough to require many hours of time and highly specialized equipment. This section addresses simplified examination techniques and screening procedures.

VISUAL ACUITY TESTING

As with any eye examination, the first step in the neuro-ophthalmic examination is to determine the patient's visual acuity. To achieve the most reliable results, measure the acuity of each eye independently with the patient wearing appropriate corrective lenses. Although using a Snellen wall chart at a distance of 20 feet is the standard method of determining acuity, using a near card in a room with good lighting will suffice in most clinical settings. Remember to make sure that patients are looking through their bifocals or reading glasses if they have them. If a patient does not have glasses, a pinhole occluder may be used to obtain a reasonable estimate of the patient's corrected visual acuity.

VISUAL FIELD TESTING

Formal evaluation of visual field (perimetry) can be time consuming and requires special training and equipment; however, confrontation field testing may be done in almost any clinical setting and provides very useful information. Each eye should be tested separately, with the patient covering 1 eye and fixating with the other on your corresponding eye. Present a random number of fingers in each of the 4 quadrants of vision, and ask the patient how many fingers are showing. It is a usually a good idea to close your other eye and make sure you can see your fingers as well. Both unilateral and bilateral peripheral field defects can be detected quickly and easily with this method.

A simple method for detecting central field defects is to ask the patient to look at a piece of graph paper or an Amsler grid. Testing each eye independently, the patient is asked to fixate on the center of the paper and to trace out areas that are missing or appear abnormal. (See Figure 3.18 in Chapter 3 for a discussion of the Amsler grid and its use in central visual field testing.) Another method of central field testing is to have the patient fixate on the examiner's nose with one eye and ask the patient if there is any part of the examiner's face that is missing or distorted. By convention, the results of visual field tests are drawn from the patient's point of view, with the left eye's field drawn on the left and right eye's field drawn on the right.

COLOR PERCEPTION AND SATURATION

Ninety percent of the fibers of the anterior visual pathways (optic nerve, chiasm, optic tracts) serve central vision. Further, central vision is extremely sensitive to the color red (the peripheral retina, by contrast, is nearly blind to the color red). Consequently, many diseases of the optic nerve and other anterior visual pathway structures will cause red hues to appear desaturated. In the office setting, pseudo-isochromatic color plates (Ishihara plates are the most popular) are a good way to test quantitatively for red and red-green color deficiencies. If acuity and visual field allow, each eye should be tested separately, and the result should be recorded as the fraction of the total number of plates that were correctly identified with each eye. It is important to note that 10% of men (and 0.4% of women) have an X-linked red-green color misperception that renders them incapable of reading pseudo-isochromatic plates correctly. Another simple, quick, and arguably more sensitive method of testing relative color saturation is the red cap test. The patient is asked to compare the color of a red bottle cap (or other bright red object) from one eye to the other. The normal eye should see the cap as a bright, saturated red; however, in an eye with optic nerve disease, the cap may appear orange, pink, or brown.

PUPILLARY EXAMINATION

Pupillary testing is a crucial part of any neuro-ophthalmic examination. Pupillary size is a function of resting autonomic tone, the light reflex, the near reflex, and local mechanical factors. Proper pupil examination requires a dim room; a small bright light source such as a bright penlight, ophthalmoscope, or transilluminator; and a distant object on which the patient may fixate. When a patient focuses on a near target, the pupils constrict due to a fixed neural relationship known as the near triad: convergence, accommodation, and pupillary constriction. (For schematic illustrations of the pupillary pathways and reflexes, see Figures 7.1 and 7.2.)

The first step in pupillary examination is to observe the resting state of the pupils in ambient room light. The pupils should be round and equal in diameter, although a difference (anisocoria) of ≤ 1 millimeter is a normal variation in up to 20% of the population. For differences of greater than 1 mm, the difference in pupil size should be recorded both in very bright and very dim lighting. Anisocoria that is more pronounced in dim lighting may indicate dysfunction of the dilating sympathetic nervous system (Horner syndrome). Anisocoria that is more pronounced in bright lighting signifies abnormal constriction and may indicate parasympathetic dysfunction (third nerve palsy, Adie tonic pupil) or pupillary trauma.

Next, test the light reflex of the pupils. In dim room lighting, shine a bright light into each pupil from either slightly below or slightly temporal to the visual axis. (Placing yourself or the light directly in front of the patient will cause the pupils to constrict due to accommodation.) There should be a brisk, simultaneous, and equal response of both pupils. For pupils that react poorly to light, it is important to test the pupil for constriction with accommodation. This is accomplished by having the patient focus with both eyes on a small, easily discernible target (such as the patient's own finger or a pen) as it is slowly moved toward the patient's face. If the pupil reacts weakly to light but strongly to accommodation, this is termed light-near dissociation and can signify an abnormality of the midbrain or ciliary ganglion.

The swinging-flashlight test is an objective and sensitive method of detecting asymmetric optic nerve disease, if performed properly. The abnormality detected with this test is the relative afferent pupillary defect (RAPD), or Marcus Gunn pupil. An RAPD is said to be present when there is a difference in the strength of the light reflex between the 2 eyes (see "Afferent Defect" in Figure 7.2). Perform the test as for the light reflex, except that the light is rhythmically swung between the 2 eyes to compare the intensity of the light reflex. It is essential that the light

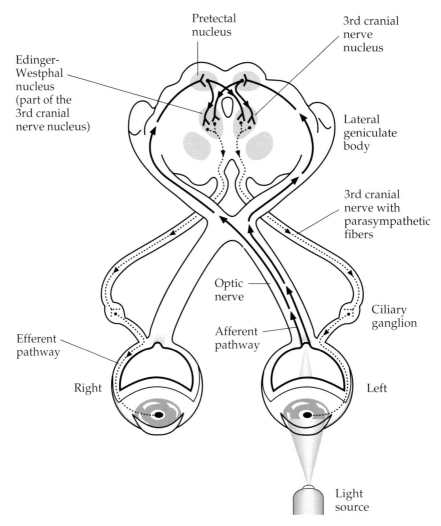

FIGURE 7.1 Pupillary pathways. This view is a cross-section. The dotted line represents the efferent pathway; the solid line represents the afferent pathway. A light stimulating the left retina generates impulses that travel up the left optic nerve and divide at the chiasm. Some impulses continue up the left tract; some cross and continue up the right tract. The impulses arrive at each pretectal nucleus and stimulate cells, which in turn send impulses down the third cranial nerve to each iris sphincter, causing each pupil to contract. It is because of the double decussation, the first in the chiasm and the second between the pretectal nuclei and the Edinger-Westphal nuclei, that the direct pupil response in the left eye equals the consensual response in the right eye.

is shone onto each eye for equal amounts of time and from the same angle. To perform the test, the light is shone into 1 eye for 3 seconds, moved rapidly across to the other eye, shone for 3 seconds, and then shifted back to the first eye. This procedure is repeated several times until the examiner is certain of the responses. Normally, the pupils should remain the same size or constrict slightly as the light is swung between the 2 eyes. An RAPD is present when there is repeatable dilation of both pupils without initial constriction as the light is swung from the normal eye to the abnormal eye.

Normal Reaction (both eyes) Efferent Defect (left eye) Afferent Defect (left eye)

Ambient light

Penlight (right eye)

Penlight (left eye)

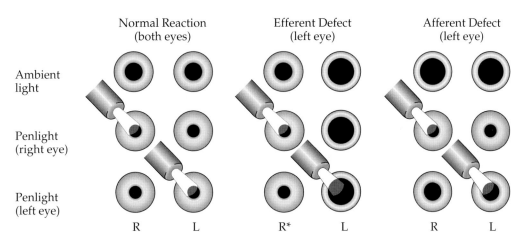

R   L   R*   L   R   L

FIGURE 7.2 Pupillary reflexes. The orientation depicted is that of the examiner looking at the patient's eyes. *Note normal constriction from consensual response.

An RAPD defect almost always indicates a lesion in the optic nerve on the affected side, although widespread or central retinal disorders may produce a subtle RAPD. Cataracts and vitreous hemorrhages generally do not affect pupillary reaction. It is important to remember 2 important points: first, since the consensual response is always balanced with the direct pupil response, an RAPD never causes anisocoria. Second, the swinging-flashlight test is a comparative test: an RAPD cannot be bilateral.

OCULAR MOTILITY TESTING

Eye movements should always be tested, especially if the patient has a complaint of double vision. Various methods are used to assess ocular alignment and motility, such as cover tests, prisms, Maddox rods, red-filters, and corneal light reflex position. For an in-depth discussion of corneal reflex and cover tests, refer to the sections "Ocular Motility Testing" in Chapter 1 and "Strabismus Testing" in Chapter 6. Very broadly, though, an examiner should be looking for the following abnormalities:

- Strabismus (abnormal ocular alignment)
- Limitation of movement of either eye
- Limitation of conjugate gaze (inability to look in a particular direction with either eye)
- Nystagmus (spontaneous to-and-fro jerking eye movements)

OPHTHALMOSCOPY

Evaluation of a patient with neurologic symptoms is not complete without evaluation of the ocular fundus. In particular, special attention should be given to the appearance of the optic disc. In some neuro-ophthalmic conditions, the optic disc may be swollen and elevated; in others, it may be pale and atrophic. The examiner should attempt to note the presence of spontaneous venous pulsations, an indication of normal intracranial pressure, as well as the presence of hemorrhage or abnormal cupping of the optic nerve.

Fundoscopy can be performed with or without pharmacologic dilation of the pupils, although dilation is preferred. Tropicamide 0.5% drops are a safe and effective agent for pupillary dilation. A common reason given by non-ophthalmologists for not dilating patients' pupils is the perceived risk of inciting angle-closure glaucoma. In fact, the risk of causing angle-closure glaucoma with pharmacologic dilation is exceedingly low. However, the physician may wish to assess anterior chamber depth before dilation.

HOW TO INTERPRET THE FINDINGS

This section reviews suggestions for evaluating the more common signs and symptoms of neuro-ophthalmic disorders.

PUPILLARY DISORDERS

Disorders of pupillary function are very helpful in localizing neurologic disease. However, concomitant ocular disease, history of ocular surgery or trauma, and the influence of systemic or local drugs on the pupils must be assessed before pupillary abnormalities can be considered neurologically significant. Some commonly encountered pupillary abnormalities are discussed below.

The Dilated Pupil

A dilated (mydriatic) pupil, especially one that does not react to light, usually indicates a loss of parasympathetic input to the iris sphincter. This may be the result of oculomotor nerve paresis, benign ciliary ganglionopathy (Adie tonic pupil), trauma to the orbital parasympathetics (traumatic mydriasis), dorsal midbrain syndrome, prior iris damage/surgery, or pharmacologic dilation.

Third Nerve Palsy

Cranial nerve III (oculomotor nerve) exerts control over the levator muscle of the eyelid and the medial rectus, inferior rectus, superior rectus, inferior oblique, and pupillary sphincter muscles. When the function of the oculomotor nerve is compromised, the eyelid becomes droopy (ptosis), the pupil dilated and poorly reactive, and the eye loses the ability to elevate, depress, or move nasally. Typically, the eye will turn outward and slightly downward. Although microvascular infarction of the nerve can occur (usually associated with diabetes and hypertension), patients with new-onset third nerve palsy should undergo emergent MRI and cerebrovascular imaging to rule out neural compression.

On the other hand, a dilated, fixed pupil in an otherwise asymptomatic, healthy patient with normal ocular motility is usually benign and may be due to migraine, Adie tonic pupil (see below), dilating agents, or secondary to previous ocular trauma.

Dorsal Midbrain Syndrome

Damage or compression of the upper brainstem can cause a characteristic cluster of ocular findings known as the dorsal midbrain (or Parinaud) syndrome. Classically, dorsal midbrain syndrome consists of loss of upgaze, convergence-retraction nystagmus (eyes briefly cross and retract with attempted upgaze), and light-near dissociation of the pupils. The patient may also exhibit eyelid retraction (Collier sign). Dorsal midbrain syndrome may be caused by hydrocephalus, a compressive lesion of the midbrain (eg, a pineal tumor), multiple sclerosis, stroke, or midbrain hemorrhage. Any patient with signs of dorsal midbrain syndrome should have an MRI.

Adie Tonic Pupil

Adie tonic pupil is a benign, idiopathic condition seen predominantly in young women and is unilateral in 80% of cases. In ordinary light, the tonic pupil is usually larger than the uninvolved pupil; the reaction to light is either diminished or absent. Reaction to accommodation, however, remains intact. Instillation of weak cholinergic agents (0.1% to 0.125% pilocarpine) will cause constriction of the involved pupil, indicating denervation hypersensitivity. By contrast, this constriction will not occur in a normal pupil. By itself, a tonic pupil is of no neurologic significance. When combined with diffuse hyporeflexia, it is called Holmes-Adie syndrome.

The Small Pupil

A small pupil in one eye that has normal reactivity and is not accompanied by other ocular abnormalities is commonly physiologic and is of no neurologic significance, particularly if the difference between the pupils is a millimeter or less. However, both Horner syndrome and tertiary syphilis must be considered.

Horner Syndrome

When accompanied by mild ptosis of the upper eyelid, a small pupil may indicate loss of sympathetic tone to the eye due to Horner syndrome (Figure 7.3). Horner syndrome is caused by dysfunction of the extensive sympathetic pathways, which extend from the posterior hypothalamus to the upper thoracic spinal cord to the

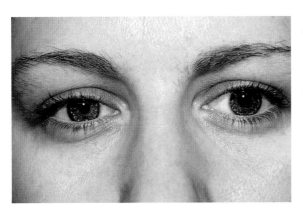

FIGURE 7.3 Horner syndrome. This acquired lesion of the cervical sympathetic chain has caused a mild ptosis of the right upper eyelid and a narrowing of the right pupil.

superior cervical ganglion and finally to the postganglionic fibers along the carotid artery and cavernous sinus (Figure 7.4). Carotid dissection, cavernous carotid aneurysm, and apical lung tumor are life-threatening lesions that can present with Horner syndrome. Patients should also be asked about any history of neck, thoracic, or spinal trauma/surgery.

Although Horner syndrome may be diagnosed by physical examination alone in most cases, examination alone may be inconclusive in some instances, and confirmatory pharmacologic testing can be helpful. This is traditionally accomplished by

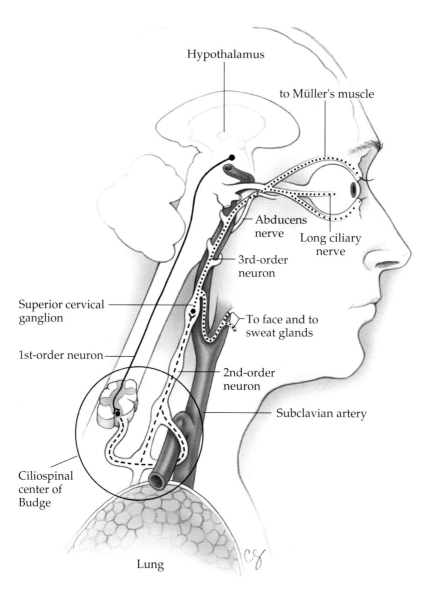

FIGURE 7.4 Anatomy of sympathetic pathway. Shown are pathways of first-order central neuron (solid line), second-order intermediate neuron (dashed line), and third-order neuron (dotted line). Note the proximity of pulmonary apex to sympathetic chain, as well as the relationship of the intracavernous sympathetic fibers to the abducens nerve. (Illustration by Christine Gralapp, MA, CMI)

the use of specially compounded cocaine and/or hydroxyamphetamine eye drops; however, increasing difficulty in obtaining these eye drops makes such tests impractical in most situations. Topical apraclonidine 0.5%, a widely available eye drop for glaucoma, is a sympathomimetic and patients with Horner syndrome will demonstrate denervation hypersensitivity to it. Instillation of apraclonidine eye drops will cause significant elevation of the eyelid and dilation of the pupil in an eye with Horner syndrome compared to the contralateral "control" eye. A reversal of anisocoria (the pupil in the abnormal eye becomes larger than its counterpart after apraclonidine is instilled) should be considered diagnostic for Horner syndrome.

Patients with Horner syndrome should have an MRI extending from the base of the brain to the mid-thoracic region. To exclude carotid artery dissection, angiography (CTA or MRA) should be performed, particularly if the Horner syndrome is acute and/or painful. Nonetheless, the majority of patients with chronic Horner syndrome ultimately will have normal imaging and are thus considered idiopathic.

Argyll Robertson Pupils

Tertiary syphilis can affect the fibers of the midbrain serving the pupillary light reflex. This may result in small, irregular pupils that demonstrate light-near dissociation. These are referred to as Argyll Robertson pupils. As is the case for dorsal midbrain syndrome, both pupils are typically involved; however, the effect may be quite asymmetric. Any patient suspected of having Argyll Robertson pupils should have serologic testing for syphilis in addition to an MRI of the brainstem.

MOTILITY DISORDERS

(It is helpful to refer to Figure 1.3, which illustrates the anatomy of the extraocular muscles.)

Evaluation of a patient complaining of double vision must include a thorough, neurologically oriented history. True binocular diplopia—double vision that involves 2 separate images, 1 of which disappears when either eye is closed—signifies strabismus acquired after the age of 7 or 8 years of age. Patients sometimes have double vision of 1 eye (monocular diplopia) that is not eliminated by occluding the fellow eye. This is usually due to refractive error, dry eye, or cataract. It is diagnostically important to note in the history whether the diplopia is binocular or monocular; transient or persistent; sudden or gradual in onset; horizontal, vertical, or diagonal; painless or painful; and whether it is the same or different in various positions of gaze.

Third Nerve Palsy

Cranial nerve III (oculomotor nerve) supplies the levator palpebrae muscle of the upper eyelid; the superior rectus, medial rectus, inferior rectus, and inferior oblique muscles; and the parasympathetic fibers to the sphincter of the iris. Complete paralysis of the oculomotor nerve produces both horizontal and vertical diplopia, with severe ptosis of the upper eyelid and an inability to move the eye inward, upward, or downward (Figure 7.5). The pupil may be dilated and nonresponsive. The most

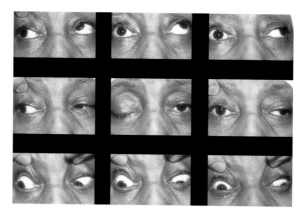

FIGURE 7.5 Third nerve palsy. The center picture shows the patient in straight-ahead gaze with a complete ptosis of the right upper lid. In the other photos, the lid is manually elevated to demonstrate the motility defect. The ocular movements are shown in the 6 cardinal positions as well as gaze up and down. Besides ptosis other obvious findings are inability to adduct or elevate the right eye. Abduction of the right eye is intact due to normal function of the sixth cranial nerve. Ocular motility of the left eye is normal. (Courtesy Steven A. Newman, MD. Reprinted from *Basic and Clinical Science Course*, Section 5: Neuro-Ophthalmology. San Francisco, CA: American Academy of Ophthalmology; 2009-2010:228.)

common causes of isolated third nerve palsy include intracranial aneurysm (especially of the posterior communicating artery), microvascular infarction within the nerve (usually associated with diabetes and hypertension), trauma, cerebral herniation, and brain tumor. Unless the clinical evidence overwhelmingly supports microvascular disease, emergent cerebral imaging with angiography must be obtained.

Fourth Nerve Palsy

Cranial nerve IV (trochlear nerve) innervates the superior oblique muscle. Complete paralysis causes vertical diplopia that is most troublesome in downgaze and contralateral sidegaze. The patient may tilt his or her head toward the opposite shoulder to minimize the diplopia. The most frequent cause of unilateral fourth nerve palsy is microvascular disease, especially associated with hypertension or diabetes. However, this is also a common congenital anomaly that can present in adulthood (Figure 7.6). The most frequent cause of bilateral fourth nerve palsy is closed head trauma.

Sixth Nerve Palsy

Cranial nerve VI (abducens nerve) supplies the lateral rectus muscle. Paralysis produces loss of abduction resulting in horizontal diplopia, with the greatest separation of images when the gaze is directed toward the affected side (Figure 7.7). Among all ages, the overall incidence of a tumor as the etiology of an isolated sixth nerve palsy is approximately 20%. Microvascular disease (increased risk with diabetes, hypertension, smoking, and hyperlipidemia) is a much more common culprit among adults, particularly in adults older than 55 years of age, in whom microvascular disease is responsible for the vast majority of sixth nerve palsies. Thus, patients

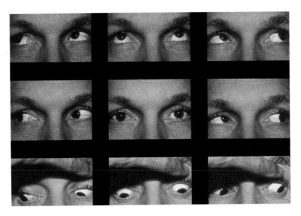

FIGURE 7.6 Fourth nerve palsy. A patient with a fourth nerve palsy complains of vertical double vision (one image above the other). In primary gaze the eyes look straight. In this patient with a right fourth nerve palsy the right hypertropia increases as the patient looks to the left. To decrease his double vision he tilts his head to the left. Tilting the head to the right (same side as the palsy) increases the double vision. (Courtesy Steven A. Newman, MD. Reprinted from *Basic and Clinical Science Course,* Section 5: Neuro-Ophthalmology. San Francisco, CA: American Academy of Ophthalmology; 2004–2005:238.)

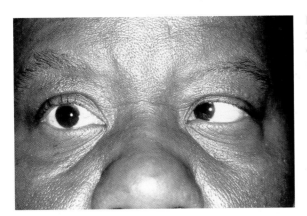

FIGURE 7.7 Sixth nerve palsy. Shown here is an impairment of abduction of the right eye on right gaze.

at risk for microvascular disease and those over 55 should initially be managed by observation, as 98% of microvascular palsies spontaneously recover within 3 to 4 months. If recovery does not ensue or if other neurologic abnormalities are present, neuroimaging is required. In adults younger than 45 years, MRI is indicated initially, as the incidence of a space-occupying lesion increases with decreasing age. Increased intracranial pressure due to pseudotumor cerebri or hydrocephalus can present infrequently with bilateral sixth nerve palsies.

For children, trauma is the most common etiology of a sixth nerve palsy (42%). Other causes in children are postviral/parainfectious disease, or inflammation of the petrous ridge from severe otitis media. Parents or caregivers should be asked about and the child should be examined for head trauma, recent systemic illness, vaccinations, and ear infections. If these are not present, or if presumed parainfectious palsy fails to recover within a few weeks, neuroimaging is indicated.

Internuclear Ophthalmoplegia

The medial longitudinal fasciculus (MLF) is a tract of internuclear neurons within the brainstem, which, among other things, carries output from the sixth nerve nuclei to the contralateral third nerve nuclei to coordinate horizontal eye movements (Figure 7.8). A lesion of the MLF interrupts this connection and manifests clinically as an internuclear ophthalmoplegia (INO). The clinical manifestations of an INO are slow and/or weak adduction of one eye and nystagmus of the abducting fellow eye in lateral gaze (Figure 7.9). An INO may be unilateral or bilateral, and the eyes may be straight in primary gaze or turned outward (exotropic). In older individuals, an internuclear ophthalmoplegia is usually due to brainstem microvascular disease and typically recovers in weeks or months. In younger adults, an INO is most commonly due to demyelinating disease, brainstem hemorrhage, or trauma. In children, an internuclear ophthalmoplegia may be due to a pontine glioma. All patients with an INO should have an MRI of the brainstem. As a rule, the diagnosis of myasthenia gravis (see below) should be considered in any patient with weak adduction, particularly if ptosis is present or there is no nystagmus of the abducting eye.

Convergence/Divergence Paresis

The ability to move the eyes together (convergence) and apart again (divergence) is important in maintaining eye alignment and fusion of images as the gaze is moved

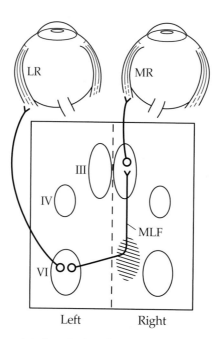

FIGURE 7.8 Internuclear ophthalmoplegia. Information travels from the sixth nerve nucleus (VI) to the ipsilateral lateral rectus muscle (LR) and, via the medial longitudinal fasciculus (MLF), to the contralateral third nerve nucleus (III) and on to the contralateral medial rectus (MR) to make both eyes turn to the side of the stimulating sixth nerve nucleus. A lesion blocking the path between the ipsilateral sixth nerve nucleus and the contralateral third nerve nucleus results in an internuclear ophthalmoplegia.

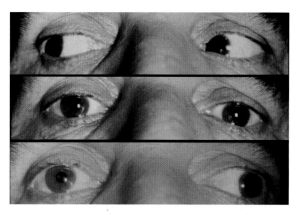

FIGURE 7.9 Unilateral right internuclear ophthalmoplegia. This 32-year-old patient with multiple sclerosis is unable to adduct the right eye on left horizontal gaze (bottom). The eyes are straight in primary gaze (middle), differentiating this condition from medial rectus underaction of intrinsic muscle or third nerve origin. (Reprinted by permission from Miller NR, ed. *Walsh & Hoyt's Clinical Neuro-Ophthalmology.* 4th ed. Vol 2. Baltimore, MD: Williams & Wilkins; 1985.)

between near and distant objects. Either of these abilities may falter with age as the consequence of chronic small vessel disease and senescent atrophy, particularly in the presence of movement disorders such as Parkinson disease.

Patients with convergence insufficiency experience double vision when viewing objects at near, but not at distance. An examination of these patients shows normal eye movement and alignment in primary gaze; however, when viewing a close object, the eyes are turned out from each other (exotropia). In contrast, people with divergence paresis experience double vision at distance but not when reading. Their motility is normal, and when measured at near, their eyes are straight; however, their eyes are crossed (esotropia) in primary distance gaze.

Myasthenia Gravis

Myasthenia gravis is a chronic autoimmune condition that interferes with neuromuscular transmission in skeletal muscles; it can affect any age and either gender. Ptosis and double vision are the presenting signs in half of the patients. Of those presenting with only ocular signs (ocular myasthenia), half will go on to develop weakness of other skeletal muscles within 2 years (generalized myasthenia). Characterized by fatigability of muscle function with sustained effort, myasthenia gravis may mimic nearly any other oculomotor paresis, including third, fourth, and sixth nerve weakness; conjugate gaze palsy; and internuclear ophthalmoplegia. As a rule, myasthenia gravis does not affect the pupil. For patients with unexplained ptosis or ocular movement problems, myasthenia gravis should always be considered.

Although the diagnosis is usually established clinically, testing for myasthenia gravis may involve serologies for acetylcholine receptor antibodies, electromyography, and the ice-pack test (temporary resolution of ptosis after an ice-pack has been placed on the eyelid for 2 minutes).

Nystagmus

Spontaneous, rhythmic, back-and-forth movement of one or both eyes is referred to as nystagmus (see "General Inspection" in Chapter 6). The direction of nystagmus may be horizontal, vertical, rotary, or a combination.

The 3 most common forms of nystagmus are benign and do not indicate central nervous system dysfunction. The first form of benign nystagmus occurs when the patient is attempting to maintain the eyes in extremes of lateral gaze. In this position, it is not unusual to see 3 to 4 "beats" of horizontal or horizontal-rotary nystagmus. End-gaze nystagmus usually dampens quickly and disappears if the patient is permitted to move the gaze slightly away from the extreme position. The second form of benign nystagmus is induced by nystagmogenic medications such as antiepileptics, barbiturates, and other sedatives. In this form, a jerk nystagmus may be present in all positions of gaze, although sustained end-gaze nystagmus is the most common form. The third form, a searching, pendular nystagmus, may be seen in individuals from birth or beginning in the first 6 months of life. This is called congenital nystagmus. Patients with congenital forms of nystagmus generally have subnormal vision and do not complain of the environment visually shaking or moving (oscillopsia).

Acquired nystagmus typically causes oscillopsia and/or vertigo and may indicate vestibular, cerebellar, or brainstem dysfunction. Representative diseases that cause nystagmus are peripheral vestibular disease, trauma, multiple sclerosis, brain tumor, and degeneration of the central nervous system. A full neurologic evaluation including an MRI is warranted for all patients with acquired nystagmus in whom peripheral vestibular disease is not clearly the cause. As a general rule, pathologic forms of nystagmus are usually detectable in the primary (straight ahead) eye position.

OPTIC NERVE DISEASE

Many disorders of the anterior visual pathways are accompanied by abnormalities of the optic nerve head. These include swelling due to increased intracranial pressure, infiltration, inflammation, and ischemia of the anterior optic nerve head; or optic nerve atrophy due to chronic optic nerve damage.

OPTIC DISC ELEVATION

Optic disc elevation is identified fundoscopically by indistinct disc margins, elevation of the optic disc, vascular tortuosity, and absence of a central cup. These features alone, however, do not distinguish pathologic disc elevation (disc edema) from congenital disc elevation. Although no single feature is reliably present or pathognomonic for acquired disc elevation, the presence of capillary hyperemia and hemorrhages on or around the disc should be considered signs of active disc edema.

Congenital Disc Elevation

Congenital disc elevation is a normal variant and may be accompanied by the presence of bright yellow, proteinaceous material within the optic disc itself (optic disc drusen). Because of its deceptive appearance, congenital fullness of the optic nerve has been referred to as pseudopapilledema (Figure 7.10, left). The condition should not be confused with true papilledema (Figure 7.10, right); however, such differentiation may be extremely difficult, requiring the assistance of an ophthalmologist and specialized testing.

Papilledema

Papilledema refers to passive swelling of the optic disc secondary to increased intracranial pressure. Funduscopic characteristics of fully developed papilledema include hyperemia of the disc, tortuosity of the veins and capillaries, blurring and elevation of the margins of the disc, obscuration of retinal vessels near the nerve, and hemorrhages on and surrounding the nerve head. Papilledema is typically bilateral, although it may be highly asymmetric. The signs of early papilledema, on the other hand, may not be obvious, with only subtle elevation of the disc margins, loss of previously identified spontaneous venous pulsations, and mild disc hyperemia. Vision is usually not affected initially; however, seconds-long graying out of vision (visual obscurations), flickering, or blurred vision may occur. Patients may also have symptoms of increased intracranial pressure, such as headache, nausea/vomiting, and/or double vision. Broadly speaking, causes of papilledema are

- Brain tumors/space-occupying lesions
- Idiopathic intracranial hypertension (pseudotumor cerebri)
- Cerebral trauma or hemorrhage
- Meningitis/encephalitis
- Dural sinus thrombosis

Any patient with suspected papilledema should have an immediate MRI or CT scan. A lumbar puncture should be performed if a mass or venous thrombosis

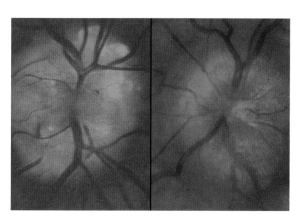

FIGURE 7.10 Pseudo-papilledema and true papilledema. On the left, pseudopapilledema from optic nerve drusen is shown; note several discrete drusen on the superior edge of the disc. On the right, true papilledema is shown; note congested capillaries and swollen nerve bundles.

has been ruled out to evaluate the cerebrospinal fluid and its pressure. Chronic papilledema can cause permanent optic nerve damage and blindness if not treated.

Passive optic disc swelling may also result from abnormal cerebral hemodynamics in malignant hypertension, anemia, and pregnancy. These forms of disc edema, although bilateral and sometimes accompanied by normal vision, do not result from increased intracranial pressure and therefore should not, strictly speaking, be termed papilledema.

Pseudotumor Cerebri

Also known as idiopathic intracranial hypertension, pseudotumor cerebri is a disorder of increased fluid pressure around the brain in the absence of a brain tumor, thrombosis, or other cerebrospinal fluid (CSF) abnormality. Most common in women between the ages of 20 and 40 who have a history of recent weight gain, the cause of pseudotumor cerebri is a subject of much debate. Venous hypertension, reduced absorption of CSF across the arachnoid granulations, and/or hormonal dysregulation are currently the top candidates.

Symptoms of pseudotumor cerebri include (in order of frequency) headache, transient blurring of vision, pulsatile tinnitus, horizontal double vision, neck stiffness, vision loss, and pain with eye movement. Signs are often limited to papilledema and occasional sixth nerve palsies. As a rule, the neurologic examination of patients with pseudotumor cerebri is otherwise normal. History of exposure to steroids, excessive vitamin A, retinoic acid, tetracycline or its derivatives, and lithium should be obtained. As for papilledema, workup includes a brain MRI followed by lumbar puncture for opening pressure and CSF profile.

Vision loss is the most dreaded consequence of pseudotumor cerebri. Chronic papilledema arising from increased intracranial pressure may result in progressive ganglion cell death as a result of compromised axonal homeostasis or ischemia. As with other optic neuropathies, visual acuity and/or visual field may be affected. Treatment of pseudotumor focuses on decreasing intracranial pressure. Weight loss, carbonic anhydrase inhibitors, CSF shunting procedures (lumboperitoneal or ventriculoperitoneal shunts), and optic nerve sheath fenestration all may be used to reduce papilledema and the risk of blindness.

Papillitis

Inflammatory edema of the disc, known as papillitis, may be indistinguishable from papilledema by its ophthalmoscopic appearance; however, clinically they are distinct. (For a comparison of papillitis and papilledema, see Figures 2.7 and 2.8.) Whereas papilledema is more commonly bilateral and vision usually remains good initially, papillitis is more commonly unilateral and is associated with decreased visual acuity, impaired color vision, visual field defects, and an afferent pupillary defect. Papillitis may result from demyelination, ischemia, infiltration, compression, or infection.

Optic Neuritis

Optic neuritis refers to inflammation and demyelination of the optic nerve. Most common in women ages 15 to 45, optic neuritis causes acute or subacute vision loss associated with periocular pain. The pain is typically exacerbated by eye movement and may precede the visual decline. Anterior optic neuritis (a form of papillitis) results in disc edema, although the swelling is typically mild. The majority of cases of optic neuritis, however, occur behind the eye (so-called *retrobulbar optic neuritis*) leaving the optic disc appearance completely normal. If the fellow optic nerve is healthy and unaffected, an afferent pupillary defect will be present. Optic neuritis frequently results in varying degrees of decreased visual acuity, impaired color vision, and visual field defects.

Optic neuritis is most commonly associated with multiple sclerosis (MS). Overall, 50% of patients presenting with isolated optic neuritis will ultimately develop MS; however, their risk is best stratified by the number of characteristic white matter lesions on an MRI (fewer lesions = lower risk). For typical optic neuritis, the vision will recover spontaneously within weeks without treatment. Intravenous corticosteroids will hasten recovery and transiently decrease the risk of recurrence, but the effects are temporary and not disease modifying. Oral corticosteroids are contraindicated as the sole treatment of optic neuritis but may be safely employed during taper from intravenous steroids. All patients with optic neuritis should have an MRI with and without contrast.

Optic neuritis may also be idiopathic, postviral, or associated with a variety of systemic conditions (eg, syphilis, sarcoidosis, collagen vascular disease, Lyme disease, HIV). All patients with optic neuritis should be evaluated by an ophthalmologist to evaluate for atypical features and a more in-depth workup.

Ischemic Optic Neuropathy

An important cause of acute vision loss in adults, ischemic optic neuropathy results from microvascular infarction of the optic nerve and presents with sudden, painless, unilateral loss of vision. The region of the optic nerve most vulnerable to ischemia is the anterior portion where it joins the eye, and ischemic damage here is referred to as anterior ischemic optic neuropathy (AION). There are 2 major variants of AION: arteritic and nonarteritic. It is critically important to differentiate the more common nonarteritic form of AION from the arteritic form because the latter is associated with giant cell (temporal) arteritis and can result in rapid bilateral blindness if not promptly treated.

Posterior ischemic optic neuropathy (PION) is much less common than AION and results in sudden, severe, unilateral or bilateral vision loss in the setting of systemic hypotension (cardiac bypass and prolonged spinal surgery being the most common settings) but can also be seen in cranial surgery, trigeminal zoster, or systemic vasculitis. The optic disc may be swollen or may appear normal.

Nonarteritic Ischemic Optic Neuropathy

Nonarteritic ischemic optic neuropathy (NAION) is the most common form of ischemic optic neuropathy and, although it can occur at any age, typically presents in patients over 40 years old who have atherosclerotic risk factors (eg, hypertension, diabetes, hyperlipidemia, smoking, sleep apnea, obesity). The pathophysiology of NAION is not well understood, although it is probably due to transient hypoperfusion of the posterior ciliary arteries supplying the optic nerve head.

Many cases of NAION occur during periods of nocturnal hypotension and present with unilateral visual loss first noted upon waking. Patients often describe loss of either the upper or lower half of their vision in the affected eye (altitudinal field loss). On examination of a patient with NAION, the visual acuity is variably affected, there is always an afferent pupillary defect (assuming the fellow eye is normal), and there is always disc edema initially. As a rule, there are no other clinical manifestations or accompanying neurologic symptoms of NAION.

There are no proven treatments and there is usually little or no recovery with NAION. Treatment is aimed at secondary prevention (treating atherosclerotic risk factors and avoiding excessive lowering of blood pressure), although there is no evidence that these measures actually reduce the risk of developing NAION in the fellow eye. All patients more than 60 years of age with suspected NAION should have an erythrocyte sedimentation rate (ESR) and a C-reactive protein (CRP) test to exclude giant cell (temporal) arteritis.

Arteritic Anterior Ischemic Optic Neuropathy

Less common than NAION, arteritic anterior ischemic optic neuropathy (AAION) is characterized by sudden, painless, and often catastrophic visual loss in patients over 60. Early recognition of AAION is critical since it is a cardinal feature of giant cell (temporal, cranial) arteritis, an idiopathic inflammatory vasculitis of the elderly that can lead to blindness, aortitis, and strokes. Although AAION often begins unilaterally, the fellow eye typically will follow rapidly, often within days, if not promptly and aggressively treated.

The most specific clinical features of giant cell arteritis include jaw claudication, new-onset headache, visual abnormalities (amaurosis fugax, diplopia, vision loss), and palpable temporal artery abnormalities (eg, decreased pulse, tenderness, or nodules). High clinical suspicion includes any 1 of these in a patient more than 60 years of age with an elevated ESR and/or CRP. The diagnosis is made by temporal artery biopsy. It is important to note that about one-fifth of patients with giant cell arteritis and vision loss have no systemic symptoms.

Treatment of AAION centers on protection of the other eye. Any patient with suspected giant cell arteritis should be started on corticosteroids immediately and scheduled for a temporal artery biopsy. Treatment should never be delayed waiting for the biopsy or its results.

Transient Monocular Blindness (Amaurosis Fugax)

Transient monocular blindness (TMB) is temporary, painless loss of vision in 1 eye and can have many causes. TMB resulting from embolic sources (amaurosis fugax) typically lasts seconds to several minutes and may affect the entire vision or only the upper or lower half. Patients over age 50 complaining of monocular visual loss lasting several minutes should be investigated for stenosis of the ipsilateral carotid artery, embolic sources of cardiac origin, and temporal arteritis. Ophthalmoscopy may be normal or reveal an intra-arterial plaque (Hollenhorst plaque) at retinal arterial bifurcations (see Figure 2.3). Evaluation of amaurosis fugax includes ESR, CRP, carotid ultrasound, and transesophageal echocardiogram. When the transient visual loss (monocular or binocular) lasts 20 to 40 minutes and is associated with photopsias (flashes of light) and/or headache, it is often due to vasospasm (migraine).

Optic Atrophy

Optic atrophy (Figure 7.11) refers to morphologic and physiologic changes of the optic nerve as a result of damage to the ganglion cells anywhere along their course (within the inner layer of the retina, the optic nerve, the optic chiasm, or the optic tract). Optic atrophy is most easily observed as a change in the appearance of the optic disc. As a result of progressive loss of axons and changes in glial tissue, the optic disc may become pale and the physiologic cup may enlarge. After extensive damage, the disc may actually appear white. Relying solely on the color of the optic nerve to diagnose optic atrophy, however, is often misleading as there is a wide range of normal coloration of the disc from person to person and from eye to eye. For example, the optic nerve usually appears paler in eyes that have undergone cataract surgery and in highly myopic eyes. A diagnosis of optic atrophy should not be made unless there is concomitant, demonstrable optic nerve dysfunction such as decreased visual acuity, visual field loss, and/or an afferent pupillary defect. Unless the cause of optic atrophy can be clearly established based on examination

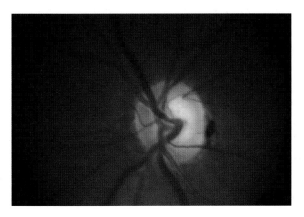

FIGURE 7.11 Optic atrophy. This left optic nerve is flat with sharp margins and a small temporal crescent of pigment (unrelated to the atrophy). Careful comparison of color of the temporal and nasal disc highlights the temporal disc pallor. (Courtesy Donald Stone, MD)

and/or history, a workup should be initiated with an orbital MRI with contrast and selected serologies. Common causes of optic atrophy include the following:

- Prior ischemic optic neuropathy
- Optic nerve compression by a mass, such as a meningioma or pituitary adenoma
- Long-standing papilledema
- Compression of the optic nerve
- Glaucoma (see Chapter 3)
- Previous ocular/optic nerve trauma
- Toxic optic neuropathy (methanol and ethambutol being most important)
- Hereditary optic neuropathies

VISUAL FIELD DEFECTS

Lesions anywhere in the visual system, from the retina to the occipital lobes, can produce visual field defects (Figure 7.12). Although there are entire texts devoted to the science of perimetry, most physicians need be concerned with only a few types of visual field loss. The following terms are commonly used to discuss visual field loss:

- Scotoma: an area of abnormal or absent vision within an otherwise intact visual field.
- Hemianopia: loss of half the visual field. Usually, this involves loss of either the right or the left half of the visual field in either eye; however, the term altitudinal hemianopia may be used to describe loss of the superior or inferior half of the visual field.
- Homonymous hemianopia: loss of either the right or the left half of the visual field in both eyes.
- Bitemporal (heteronymous) hemianopia: loss of the temporal half of the visual field in both eyes. A binasal hemianopia, although technically possible, is exceedingly rare and usually not due to neurologic disease. Neurologically significant field defects are most often central scotomas (due to optic nerve or retinal lesions), bitemporal field defects (due to chiasmal disease), or homonymous visual field defects (due to retrochiasmal damage to the optic tracts, the radiations, or the occipital cortex).

Lesions anterior to the chiasm (within the optic nerve itself) produce visual field defects in the ispilateral eye only. These defects are typically a central scotoma or altitudinal hemianopia, with accompanying afferent pupillary defect. Common causes of unilateral optic neuropathy include optic neuritis/papillitis, optic nerve glioma, meningioma, and ischemic optic neuropathy.

Lesions affecting the optic chiasm itself produce visual field defects that affect both eyes, but in a dissimilar fashion. The most common example is a bitemporal hemianopia caused by pituitary adenoma, craniopharyngioma, or parasellar

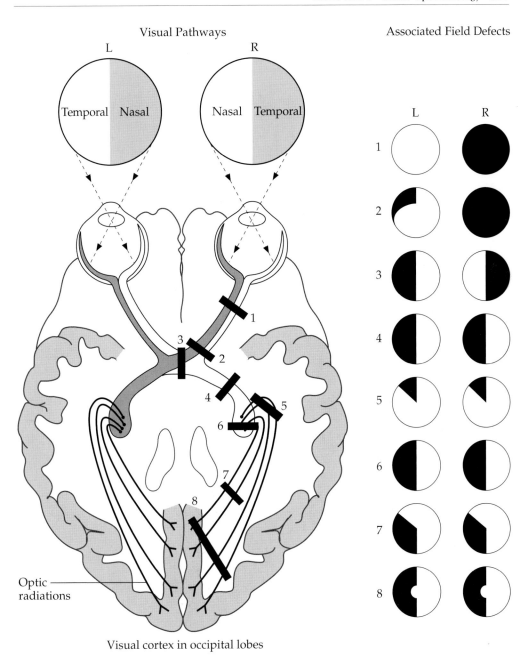

Visual Pathways   Associated Field Defects

FIGURE 7.12 Visual pathways with associated field defects. For the visual pathways, the view shown is a cross-section seen from above. Note that objects in the right half of the visual field form images in the left half of each retina and are transmitted to the left hemisphere. The numbers correspond to lesions in the visual pathways and to the field defects that result from these interruptions. For the purposes of the diagram, the fields shown reflect the effects of total interruption of the indicated structures. In actuality, partial impairment is more the rule than the exception. The key at the top of the next page indicates the site of each lesion and the associated field defect.

SITE OF LESION	ASSOCIATED FIELD DEFECT
1 Optic nerve	Monocular loss of vision
2 Optic nerve merging with chiasm	Monocular loss of vision associated with contralateral impairment of temporal field
3 Optic chiasm	Bitemporal hemianopia
4 Optic tract	Total homonymous hemianopia (usually noncongruous if incomplete)
5 Temporal lobe	Upper homonymous hemianopia
6 Geniculate body	Rare total homonymous hemianopia
7 Parietal lobe	Lower homonymous quadrantanopia
8 Occipital lobe	Variety of homonymous hemianopias, ranging from total to small homonymous scotomas, depending on the portion of lobe involved; high degree of congruity

meningioma. Another visual field defect due to a parasellar mass is loss of central field in one eye and a temporal visual field defect in the other eye, which is referred to as a junctional scotoma.

Lesions affecting the visual pathways behind the chiasm produce a homonymous hemianopia. Because the fibers serving the corresponding portions of the 2 retinas lie increasingly closer together as the fibers pass back toward the occipital cortex, there is greater correspondence of the field defects between the 2 eyes as the lesion is located more posteriorly. Central visual acuity is not affected in homonymous hemianopias unless both hemispheres are involved. Stroke is the most common cause of a homonymous hemianopia, followed by trauma and mass lesions. Middle cerebral artery occlusion tends to cause a complete hemianopia with other neurologic signs, whereas posterior cerebral artery occlusion causes neurologically isolated homonymous hemianopias.

VISUAL HALLUCINATIONS

Although visual hallucinations may occur for many reasons (migraine, seizure, delirium, dementia, psychosis, or pharmacologic agents), the most common cause of visual hallucinations is Charles Bonnet syndrome (CBS). CBS is characterized by release hallucinations that occur in cognitively intact individuals with bilaterally decreased vision. The hallucinations of the syndrome are typically of colorful geometric patterns, faces, animals, flowers, or people. As a rule, these hallucinations are solely visual, sporadic, and not associated with other neurologic or cognitive deficits. CBS has been described in over 15% of patients with vision worse than 20/80 in both eyes. CBS has also been described in patients with bilateral visual field defects but normal acuities. The hallucinations of CBS are believed to be release phenomenon from the visual associative cortex and are more common in elderly patients. Visual hallucinations in the setting of normal acuities and visual fields should raise the possibility of early dementia, particularly Lewy body dementia, or other neurologic disease. Although simple reassurance of patients is all that is needed in most cases, improved lighting at home and increased social interactions may be helpful. Pharmacologic treatment (with atypical antipsychotics or antidepressants) is rarely needed.

COGNITIVE VISUAL LOSS: THE VISUAL VARIANT OF ALZHEIMER'S DISEASE

Elderly patients or their family may complain that the patient cannot see or read well, although eye exams are repeatedly normal. Many of these patients have had multiple eye exams and may have purchased several new pairs of glasses or even undergone cataract surgery. Often, these patients are suffering from early dementia and have difficulty with poor object recognition and simultagnosia (an inability to concentrate on more than one visual stimulus at the same time), such that they can read individual letters but cannot group letters into words or words into sentences. Because of expanding and progressive cortical and subcortical dysfunction, they may also demonstrate homonymous visual field defects without a clear correlate on cerebral imaging.

An easy way to test for visual dementia is by a clock drawing. The patient is given a circle and asked to draw the numbers and hands of a clock with the time at 10 minutes after 11 o'clock. There are many ways to grade the results, but abnormal clock drawing is both sensitive and specific in identifying dementia. These patients should be referred for neuropsychiatric testing and a geriatrics or neurology consultation.

POINTS TO REMEMBER

- Testing of visual acuity, pupils, and visual fields is critical in the evaluation of the abnormal optic disc.
- A patient with a unilateral optic nerve lesion should have equal pupils in ambient light but an abnormal swinging-flashlight test.
- A blurred disc margin is not diagnostic for papilledema. Other signs and symptoms must be considered.
- Chiasmal disease is most likely to cause a bitemporal field defect and is usually due to a benign neoplasm.
- If one of the following is abnormal—pupil, lid position, or ocular motility— look closely for involvement of the others.
- Cranial nerves V and VII should be checked if ocular motility is abnormal and cranial nerve palsy is suspected.
- Slowly progressive vision loss or cranial nerve palsy should prompt consideration of a compressive lesion such as a tumor or aneurysm.
- Abrupt visual loss or diplopia implies vascular disease. Do not forget to consider giant cell arteritis in patients over 60.

SAMPLE PROBLEMS

1. A 45-year-old woman comes to the emergency center because of severe left-sided headache and double vision that began the night before, immediately following vigorous exercise. As you examine her, she continues to complain of severe left-sided headache. Her neuro-ophthalmologic examination is normal, except that the left upper lid is ptotic (droopy); and the left pupil is dilated 3 mm more than the right and responds very poorly to light. Her motility looks grossly normal. What is your differential diagnosis? How would you proceed with evaluation and management?

   Answer: Despite the grossly normal ocular motility, the ptosis of the eyelid combined with pupil dilation and subjective diplopia are consistent with early left third nerve palsy. The features of this case—including the age and gender of the patient, the suddenness of onset, the accompanying headache, and the fact that onset occurred in conjunction with vigorous exercise—require consideration of an aneurysm of the circle of Willis. Such an aneurysm is the most common cause of third nerve palsy with pupillary involvement. This is one of the true ophthalmic emergencies. The management in this case calls for immediate cerebrovascular imaging and a neurosurgical consultation.

   On the other hand, a pupil-sparing third nerve palsy is not a neurosurgical emergency, and the patient should be worked up for diabetes, syphilis, and other vascular disease. It is important to note that a third nerve palsy can be considered pupil-sparing only if the palsy is complete and the pupil is totally normal.

2. A 25-year-old medical student suddenly complains of horizontal diplopia. Her eyes are straight when looking directly ahead, but when she attempts to look to the right or left, the adducting eye fails to move normally. She also exhibits horizontal nystagmus of the abducting eye. What is the neuro-anatomic localization of this problem? What is the etiologic diagnosis?

   Answer: The description is that of bilateral internuclear ophthalmoplegia. The medial longitudinal fasciculi conduct impulses to the third cranial nerve nuclei essential for coordinated horizontal eye movements. Acute, bilateral impairment of function of the medial longitudinal fasciculi occurring in this age group is typical of multiple sclerosis.

3. A 32-year-old geologist has noticed slowly progressive blurring of vision for about a month. An optometrist changed her prescription, but the new glasses were of minimal benefit. After the symptom had been present for 3 months, she visited her family doctor, who found nothing wrong and referred her to a neurologist. The neurologist could find no abnormality and suggested she might be suffering from stress. She has now come to the emergency center because

her vision has become distressingly blurred. You conduct a basic eye examination and find the following: visual acuity in the left eye is 20/60 and does not improve with a pinhole lens, while the right eye is normal; the swinging-flashlight test discloses a left RAPD; a confrontation visual field test suggests a visual field defect in the left eye only; and ophthalmoscopy reveals mild pallor of the left optic disc. What is the differential diagnosis? Is additional testing required at this time, or should the patient merely be observed further?

Answer: The history of slowly progressive visual loss and the presence of an RAPD are evidence of a left optic nerve lesion. Optic neuritis is a possibility, but it usually produces sudden onset of visual loss, with recovery after a few weeks or months. The history and the findings are strongly suggestive of a tumor compressing the left optic nerve. Detailed visual field testing will probably reveal a major field defect in the left eye and a normal field in the right eye. This localizes the lesion to the prechiasmal optic nerve, either in the orbit or in the brain. A CT scan or an MRI with and without gadolinium would be the test to order next, with the expectation that it will show a meningioma or another kind of mass compressing the optic nerve.

4. A patient cannot see in the temporal visual field in either eye. Which one of the following findings is most likely to be associated with this defect?

    a. Tilted optic discs
    b. Pituitary tumor
    c. Neurofibromatosis
    d. Optic nerve toxicity
    e. Infarction

    Answer: b. The fact that the field loss respects the vertical meridian in each eye localizes the pathology to the optic chiasm. Pituitary tumor is the most common cause of a chiasmal syndrome. Tilted optic discs can produce temporal field loss, but the defects would extend only up to the blind spot and not to the vertical meridian. Neurofibromatosis can be associated with chiasmal glioma, but pituitary tumor is a more common association. This is not the picture of optic nerve toxicity, which is typically characterized by bilateral central scotomas with intact peripheral fields. Infarction rarely occurs in the chiasm.

5. A 64-year-old woman reports progressive onset of ptosis and diplopia over an 8-month period. On examination, the left eye is normal but the right eye reveals 4 mm of ptosis, limitation of eye movement in all directions, a smaller 4 mm pupil that does not react to light or dilate in darkness, and loss of corneal sensation. Which of the following is the most likely diagnosis?

    a. Myasthenia gravis
    b. Graves ophthalmopathy
    c. Intracavernous meningioma

d. Aneurysm of the posterior communicating artery

e. Glioma of the right midbrain

Answer: c. The patient's findings can best be explained by involvement of the third, fifth, sixth, and sympathetic nerves. Fourth nerve involvement cannot be determined from the description. A mid-dilated pupil that does not react to light or dilate in darkness usually indicates impairment of both the parasympathetic and the sympathetic innervation of the pupil. This finding as well as the other findings can best be explained by a lesion in the cavernous sinus. Meningioma and internal carotid artery aneurysm are the most common causes, particularly with a history of slow progression. Myasthenia gravis and Graves ophthalmopathy would not produce the pupillary or sensory findings noted in this patient. An aneurysm of the posterior communicating artery could produce a third nerve palsy but would not be expected to produce the other findings. A midbrain lesion typically produces bilateral ptosis, if any, and could not explain the sensory findings.

6. A 75-year-old woman presents complaining of difficulty with reading. She has had several eye examinations and has purchased 3 new pairs of glasses, with similar prescriptions from different physicians, none of which have helped. Her visual acuity on testing is 20/25 OU, and her confrontation visual fields are normal. The remainder of her ophthalmic exam is normal.

A. Which is the most appropriate next step in your evaluation?

a. Perform a visual spatial examination, such as drawing a clock face or copying intersecting pentagons, to evaluate her for signs of early dementia.

b. Refer her for a manifest refraction, cycloplegic refraction, and postcycloplegic refraction to confirm that the glasses are correct.

c. Refer her to optometry for eye exercises and vision therapy for possible dyslexia.

d. Reassure the patient that she has good acuity and peripheral vision, and follow up with her in 1 year.

Answer: a. Early dementia may present with simultagnosia, or difficulty with the presentation of multiple stimuli simultaneously. This can be seen in patients who can see but not read, as the multiple letters forming words, or multiple words forming sentences, overwhelm their cognitive functioning. An additional test is to show the patient an advertisement in a magazine and ask him or her to describe what is happening. The patient may be able to identify different items in the picture but not put the items together into the story that the advertiser is trying to promote. A more complete evaluation can be performed through neuropsychology testing and neurologic consultation.

B. The same patient is due to renew her driver's license this month and wants the motor vehicle form filled out. What is the best test to evaluate this patient's risk of motor vehicle accident and assess her ability to drive?

   a. Visual acuity test

   b. Visual field test

   c. Useful field of view evaluation

   d. Dilated fundus examination

Answer: c. Evaluation of the useful field of view tests the patient's ability to react to briefly presented peripheral visual stimuli while attending to a central visual target. Difficulty in passing this test has been correlated with an increased risk of motor vehicle accident, as well as with bodily injury to the patient and to others. It should be considered for patients with signs of dementia and difficulty with visual processing. Although not currently widely available, the useful field of view test may be found at local neurology, low vision, and ophthalmology departments in teaching facilities.

ANNOTATED RESOURCES

Glaser JS. *Neuro-Ophthalmology.* 2nd ed. Philadelphia, PA: JB Lippincott Co; 1999. This is an excellent, readable reference in neuro-ophthalmology, concise yet thorough.

Kline LB, Bajandas FJ. *Neuro-Ophthalmology Review Manual.* 6th ed. Thorofare, NJ: SLACK Incorporated; 2008. Excellent, concise review of neuro-ophthalmology with outstanding diagrams and tables.

Lee AG, Beaver HA, Jogerst G, et al. Screening elderly patients in an outpatient ophthalmology clinic for dementia, depression, and functional impairment. *Ophthalmology.* 2003;110:651–657.

Miller NR, Newman NJ, eds. *Walsh & Hoyt's Clinical Neuro-Ophthalmology.* 6th ed. Philadelphia, PA: Lippincott Williams & Wilkins; 2004. This multivolume set is the complete reference for clinical neuro-ophthalmology—the encyclopedia on the subject. Most important, it contains a thorough review of the literature.

Movaghar MD, Lawrence MG. "Eye Exam: The Essentials." In: *The Eye Examination and Ophthalmic Instruments.* San Francisco. CA: American Academy of Ophthalmology; 2001, reviewed for currency in 2007. Three titles on the DVD provide the basic framework for the ocular examination of an adult or child, as well as the use of common ophthalmic instruments.

Schadlu AP, Schadlu R, Shepherd JB 3rd. Charles Bonnet syndrome: a review. *Curr Opin Ophthalmol.* 2009;20:219–222.

Spalton DJ, Hitchings RA, Hunter PA, eds. *Atlas of Clinical Ophthalmology*. 3rd ed. St Louis, MO: Mosby-Year Book, 2004. The neuro-ophthalmology section in this atlas is very good.

Trobe JD. *The Physician's Guide to Eye Care*. 3rd ed. San Francisco, CA: American Academy of Ophthalmology; 2006. This brief but comprehensive and well-illustrated resource covers the principal clinical ophthalmic problems that nonophthalmologist physicians are likely to encounter, organized for practical use by practitioners.

Ocular Manifestations of Systemic Disease

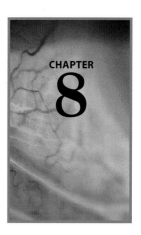

OBJECTIVES

As a primary care physician, you should be aware that many systemic diseases have ocular signs and symptoms that may result in serious ocular sequelae. You should become familiar with the important features of several of these conditions, including diabetes mellitus, hypertension, sickle cell anemia, thyroid disease, sarcoidosis and other inflammatory and autoimmune conditions, malignancy, acquired immunodeficiency syndrome, syphilis, and other systemic infections. Issues around pregnancy are also noted. To achieve these objectives, you should learn to

➤ Perform a thorough eye examination (see Chapter 1)
➤ Recognize the characteristic features, especially the ophthalmoscopic features, of these diseases
➤ Determine when it is appropriate to refer a patient to an ophthalmologist for consultation or treatment

RELEVANCE

Recognition of the ocular signs, symptoms, and complications of many systemic diseases is vitally important for good medical practice. As an example, diabetes mellitus affects more than 18 million Americans and is the leading cause of blindness in working-age Americans. Treatment of diabetic retinopathy is directed toward the prevention of visual loss. Several national clinical trials sponsored by the National Eye Institute have demonstrated that with appropriate referral and treatment the incidence of severe visual loss can be reduced by at least 90%. Because ocular findings may reflect disease progression, regular ophthalmologic examination can be beneficial in initiating or modifying treatment in a timely fashion.

DIABETES MELLITUS

Diabetes may have various ocular complications including refractive changes and cataract formation, but the most important is retinopathy. The longer a person suffers from diabetes, the greater the likelihood of developing diabetic retinopathy. Five years after diagnosis, 23% of patients with insulin-dependent diabetes mellitus (IDDM, type 1) have diabetic retinopathy; after 15 years, 80% have retinopathy; and after 20 years, 50% have the most severe subtype, proliferative diabetic retinopathy.

Diabetic patients who have non–insulin-dependent diabetes mellitus (NIDDM, type 2) have a similar but slightly lower prevalence of retinopathy. Because patients with type 2 diabetes may not be diagnosed until years after onset of their disease, many patients already have significant retinopathy at the time of diagnosis, especially certain demographic groups such as the Hispanic population.

The Diabetes Control and Complications Trial (DCCT) showed that intensive glycemic control is associated with a reduced risk of newly diagnosed retinopathy and reduced progression of existing retinopathy in people with IDDM. Furthermore, the DCCT showed that intensive glycemic control (median A1C was 7%), compared to conventional treatment (median A1C was 9%), was associated with reduction in progression to severe nonproliferative and proliferative retinopathy, a decreased incidence of macular edema, and reduction in need for panretinal and focal macular laser photocoagulation.

The Epidemiology of Diabetes Interventions and Complications (EDIC) study showed that the benefits of tight glycemic control were long lasting. The United Kingdom Prospective Diabetes Study (UKPDS) demonstrated similar outcomes in type 2 diabetics and, in addition, found that tight blood pressure control was as important as tight glycemic control in preventing the development and progression of diabetic retinopathy.

Advanced diabetic retinopathy is associated with cardiovascular disease risk factors. Patients with proliferative diabetic retinopathy are also at increased risk of heart attack, stroke, diabetic nephropathy, amputation, and death. The results of the DCCT showed that the lowering of blood glucose reduces ocular complications as well as other microvascular complications, such as nephropathy and neuropathy. It is important that all patients with diabetes are educated about the importance of determining and maintaining glycosylated hemoglobin levels to improve glycemic control.

The initial stage of the ocular disease is called *nonproliferative diabetic retinopathy* (NPDR), the first manifestation of which is microaneurysm formation. Capillaries leak and later become occluded. The retinal findings of mild and moderate NPDR also include dot-and-blot hemorrhages, hard exudates, cotton-wool spots (infarctions of the nerve fiber layer), and macular edema (Figures 8.1 and 8.2). Diabetic macular edema (DME), present in 5% to 15% of diabetic patients, is the most common cause of visual impairment in diabetic retinopathy.

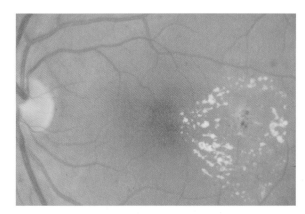

FIGURE 8.1 Nonproliferative diabetic retinopathy with clinically significant macular edema. Left macula with scattered microaneurysms and a small ring of exudate originating from small clusters of microaneurysms above the right fovea. Vascular leakage has also resulted in macular edema that cannot be visualized in this photograph. (Courtesy Stephen Fransen, MD)

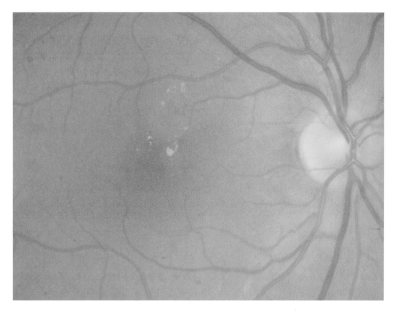

FIGURE 8.2 Nonproliferative diabetic retinopathy. Right macula with small retinal hemorrhages and ring exudates temporal to the right fovea. Prior focal laser treatment has been applied to the microaneurysms in the center of the ring. The ring will take months to resolve completely. (Courtesy Stephen Fransen, MD)

Some eyes may eventually progress to severe NPDR, which heralds the onset of the most serious form of retinopathy, the proliferative stage. Severe NPDR, or preproliferative retinopathy, is marked by increased vascular tortuosity and hemorrhagic activity, venous beading, and widespread intraretinal microvascular abnormalities (Figure 8.3). Of patients diagnosed with severe NPDR, 40% will develop proliferative diabetic retinopathy within 1 year.

Proliferative diabetic retinopathy (PDR) is the leading cause of blindness in diabetics. As a response to continued retinal ischemia, new blood vessels (neovascularization) grow over the optic disc (NVD) or elsewhere (NVE) on the retinal surface (Figures 8.4 and 8.5). Neovascularization can also occur on the surface of the iris (rubeosis iridis or NVI), causing severe glaucoma.

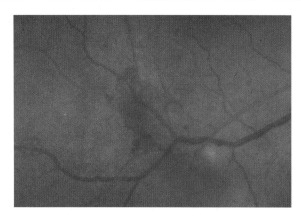

FIGURE 8.3 Early proliferative diabetic retinopathy. Venous beading (irregular caliber) along retinal vein with cotton-wool spots and neovascularization elsewhere (NVE). More subtle findings include preretinal hemorrhage and microscopic vitreous hemorrhage. (Courtesy Stephen Fransen, MD)

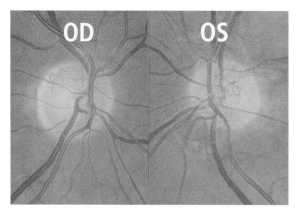

FIGURE 8.4 Proliferative diabetic retinopathy. These photographs are from the same patient. The right optic nerve has 2 new vessels over the superior aspect of the optic nerve. The left optic nerve has more advanced neovascularization. To prevent progression of the neovascularization and possible vitreous hemorrhage, panretinal photocoagulation is required. Early diagnosis and treatment of neovascularization is important to prevent visual disability. (Courtesy Cynthia A. Bradford, MD)

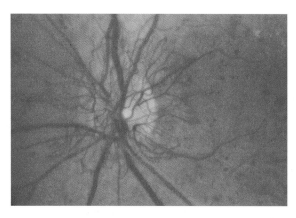

FIGURE 8.5 Proliferative diabetic retinopathy. Shown here is more advanced neovascularization of the optic nerve. These new vessels proliferate and extend into the vitreous. Later diagnosis and treatment can be more costly due to greater need for surgical intervention and is also associated with greater visual impairment and disability.

If an eye with proliferative retinopathy is not treated, these fragile new vessels can bleed into the vitreous. Fibrous tissue that accompanies the new vessels will contract and may cause a traction retinal detachment. Once these severe blinding complications (vitreous hemorrhage or traction retinal detachment) have occurred, vitrectomy with laser surgery may be necessary in the attempt to restore vision.

PDR and DME may remain asymptomatic well beyond the optimal stage for treatment. All patients with diabetes should be referred to an ophthalmologist for examination and annual follow-up. Detection of treatable macular edema and proliferative retinopathy requires stereoscopic biomicroscopy and indirect ophthalmoscopy through dilated pupils. Examination with the handheld direct ophthalmoscope is not nearly sufficient to rule out significant, treatable diabetic retinopathy. All patients with nonproliferative and proliferative retinopathy require frequent ophthalmoscopic examinations, and some require specialized examination techniques such as fluorescein angiography and optical coherence tomography (OCT) to more precisely identify ischemia and leakage and to guide therapy.

Eyes with clinically significant macular edema (CSME), DME that involves or is threatening the fovea, will require laser surgery (focal treatment) to areas of leaking blood vessels. This treatment has been demonstrated to reduce visual loss by approximately 50%. Antiangiogenic therapy (eg, intravitreal ranibizumab therapy) may also be effective in reducing DME and improving vision.

In treating proliferative retinopathy, the ophthalmologist scatters 1000 to 2000 laser burns or more under the surface of the retina well away from the posterior pole (Figure 8.6). This treatment is based on the concept that a reduction of the metabolic oxygen requirement of the retina or destruction of vascular endothelial growth factor (VEGF)-secreting cells promotes regression of the neovascular tissue.

Many patients require frequent panretinal photocoagulation (PRP) laser treatments when the disease is actively progressing. Appropriately timed effective PRP surgery can reduce the incidence of severe visual loss by at least 50% and as much as 90%. Local ranibizumab (Lucentis) therapy with intravitreal injections may also be effective.

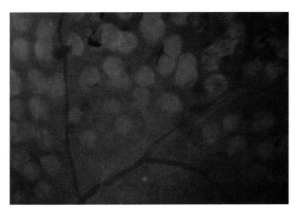

FIGURE 8.6 Panretinal argon laser photocoagulation. Shown here are old argon laser burns in a diabetic patient with proliferative retinopathy. Initially the burns are white, but with time they develop variable pigmentation from chorioretinal scarring.

Type 1 diabetics should be screened by an ophthalmologist once they are post-pubertal and have had diabetes mellitus for 5 years or longer. All individuals with type 2 diabetes should be examined at the time of diagnosis, as a subset will have retinopathy at baseline, especially in high-risk demographic groups such as the Hispanic population. More frequent examinations are required for patients who have poor glycemic control, hypertension, proteinuria, or anemia, as they are at higher risk for more rapid progression of their retinopathy.

Patients who have already been treated with laser surgery or vitrectomy should adhere to a follow-up schedule determined by their ophthalmologist. It is not unusual to require additional treatment. Women with type 1 diabetes who are, or plan to become, pregnant should be examined by an ophthalmologist preconception or during the first trimester. They may need further examinations if baseline retinopathy is present because pregnancy can severely exacerbate diabetic retinopathy.

HYPERTENSION

To understand the effects of systemic hypertension on the retinal vasculature, it is helpful to divide hypertensive retinopathy into 2 classifications: changes due to arteriolar sclerosis and changes due to elevated blood pressure.

ARTERIOLAR SCLEROSIS

Although aging causes thickening and sclerosis of the arterioles, prolonged systemic hypertension (usually diastolic pressure greater than 100 mm Hg) accelerates this process. Thickening of the walls of the retinal arterioles results in characteristic ophthalmoscopic features of retinal arteriolar sclerosis: an increase in the light reflex of the arteriole and changes in arteriovenous (A/V) crossing. The amount of arteriolar sclerosis depends on the duration and severity of the hypertension and may reflect the condition of the arterioles elsewhere in the body.

In a normal eye, the retinal arterioles are transparent tubes with blood visible by ophthalmoscopy; a light streak is reflected from the convex wall of the arteriole. As arteriolar sclerosis causes thickening of the vessel wall, the central light reflex increases in width. After sclerosis progresses, the light reflex occupies most of the width of the vessels; at this point, the vessels are called *copper-wire arterioles*. As sclerosis continues, the light reflex is obscured totally. These arterioles appear whitish and are referred to as *silver-wire arterioles*.

Because the arterioles and veins share a common sheath within the retinal tissue at crossing sites, A/V crossing changes can be viewed (Figure 8.7). The vein may be elevated or depressed by the arteriole and, in more severe cases, may undergo an abrupt right-angle change in course just as it reaches the arteriole.

Alterations in the caliber of the vein may occur because of compression and constriction at the A/V crossing (ie, nicking), resulting in dilation of the distal portion of the vein and tapering of the vein on either side of the artery. All of these A/V crossing changes are most significant when found at or beyond the second bifurcation of the arteriole, which is about 1 disc diameter distal to the optic nerve head.

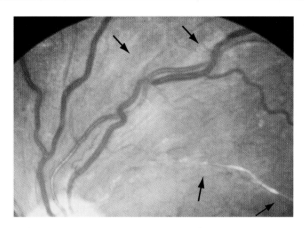

FIGURE 8.7 Hypertensive retinopathy in a patient with long-standing hypertension. Notice a single retinal vessel with areas of copper wiring and silver wiring (lower arrows). A/V crossing changes are also visible as an abrupt right-angle change of a vein at the first A/V crossing, and nicking of the vein at the second A/V crossing (upper arrows).

Severe A/V nicking can lead to branch retinal vein occlusion (BRVO), which will appear as diffuse retinal hemorrhages and cotton-wool spots in the sector of the retina that is drained by the affected vein. If accompanied by macular edema, central visual acuity may be decreased and laser treatment may be necessary in certain cases. If retinal ischemia is present, patients are at risk for neovascularization and vitreous hemorrhage, which may also benefit from laser therapy.

Unlike BRVO, branch retinal artery occlusion (BRAO) and central retinal artery occlusion (CRAO) are usually the result of systemic embolism from the carotid system in patients older than the age of 50 and from the cardiac system in those under the age of 50. Retinal artery occlusions are associated with ischemic whitening of the retina, and in the case of a CRAO, a cherry-red spot may be present due to foveal perfusion by the underlying choroid.

Older patients with CRAO should be screened for symptoms and signs of giant cell arteritis. Emergent sedimentation rate (ESR) and C-reactive protein (CRP) tests should be obtained and temporal artery biopsy should be considered if GCA is suspected; systemic prednisone may prevent blindness in the fellow eye.

ELEVATED BLOOD PRESSURE

A moderate acute rise in blood pressure results in constriction of the arterioles. A severe acute rise in blood pressure (usually diastolic pressure greater than 120 mm Hg and systolic pressure greater than 200 mm Hg) causes fibrinoid necrosis of the vessel wall, resulting in exudates, cotton-wool spots, flame-shaped hemorrhages, and even subretinal fluid. In the most severe form of hypertensive retinopathy, malignant hypertension (Figure 8.8), the optic disc swelling that occurs resembles the swelling seen in papilledema, and exudates can assume a stellate configuration in the outer plexiform layer of Henle referred to as a *macular star*.

DIAGNOSTIC CONCERNS

The relationship between hypertensive vascular changes and the changes of arteriosclerotic vascular disease is complex, with great variation in the expression of these disease processes. Hence, classification of retinal vascular changes caused

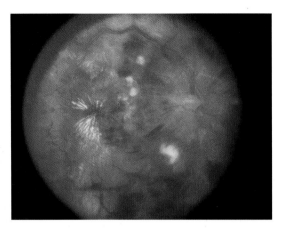

FIGURE 8.8 Malignant hypertension. This figure demonstrates ocular findings associated with severe hypertension. Note the disc edema, macular exudates, intraretinal hemorrhage with nerve fiber layer infarct, and venous congestion. (Courtesy Harry W. Flynn Jr, MD. Reprinted from *Basic and Clinical Science Course*, Section 12: Retina and Vitreous. San Francisco, CA: American Academy of Ophthalmology; 2010–2011:111.)

strictly by hypertension is difficult. One commonly used system is the Modified Scheie Classification of Hypertensive Retinopathy:

- Grade 0: No changes
- Grade 1: Barely detectable arterial narrowing
- Grade 2: Obvious arterial narrowing with focal irregularities
- Grade 3: Grade 2 plus retinal hemorrhages and/or exudates
- Grade 4: Grade 3 plus disc swelling

Hypertension is also associated with BRAO, BRVO, CRVO, and retinal arterial macroaneurysms. In order of importance, the most sensitive ophthalmoscopic indicators of hypertension are attenuation of the retinal arterioles, focal narrowing, and A/V crossing changes.

MANAGEMENT

The primary goal in managing systemic hypertension is adequate control of the blood pressure to preserve the integrity of the cerebral, cardiac, and renal circulations. A sudden, severe increase in blood pressure also can compromise the retinal and choroidal circulations, resulting in loss of vision or visual field. Under these circumstances, the blood pressure should be lowered in a controlled fashion because a sudden drop in tissue perfusion could result in optic nerve infarction and permanent loss of vision. In chronic hypertension control avoid giving the antihypertensive medication at night before sleep. Monitoring blood pressure for 24 hours has shown a natural, nocturnal drop in blood pressure, which may be compounded by the patient's antihypertensive regimen and may lead to ischemic optic neuropathy or worsening of glaucomatous visual field loss.

PREGNANCY

Although pregnancy is not a disease, it can cause numerous changes in the functioning and health of the eye. Several physiologic changes occur that are not considered pathologic. These include lowering of the intraocular pressure, decrease in corneal sensitivity, and transient loss of accommodation. Pregnant women frequently suffer from dry eyes and can experience changes in their refractive error. Therefore, pregnant patients should be discouraged from changing their prescriptions for glasses or contact lenses until after delivery. In the early postpartum period and while breast feeding, the patient should not have corneal refractive surgery performed.

In addition to physiologic changes, pathologic ocular conditions may occur during pregnancy. There is an increased incidence of central serous chorioretinopathy and uveal melanomas in pregnant versus nonpregnant women. Pregnancy-induced hypertension can cause visual disturbances such as scotoma, diplopia, and dimness of vision. Visual changes may be a sign of impending seizure in a preeclamptic patient. Retinal vascular changes can occur in toxemia, including focal and generalized arteriolar narrowing. Although uncommon, hemorrhages, exudates, diffuse retinal edema, and papilledema may appear. Serous exudative retinal detachments occur in 10% of patients with eclampsia.

Preexisting conditions such as diabetic retinopathy can also be affected by pregnancy. All pregnant diabetics should have a baseline exam in the first trimester. Those without retinopathy are unlikely to develop it during their pregnancy. Patients who have background diabetic retinopathy at the beginning of their pregnancy often have worsening of the retinopathy during the second trimester, which may improve in the third trimester and postpartum period. It is recommended that an ophthalmologist see these patients at least once per trimester. Proliferative retinopathy frequently progresses during pregnancy and needs to be monitored closely by an ophthalmologist as laser intervention may be necessary, although there are reports of reversible DME and PDR after delivery. Women with gestatimal diabetes are not at risk for retinopathy.

SICKLE CELL ANEMIA

Patients with sickle hemoglobin C (SC) and sickle cell thalassemia (S Thal) disease are more likely to have ocular involvement due to sickle cell than patients with sickle cell (SS) disease. Intravascular sickling, hemolysis, hemostasis, and then thrombosis lead to arteriolar occlusion followed by capillary nonperfusion. As with diabetes, inadequate perfusion of the retina can stimulate retinal neovascularization, which is typically more peripheral and can lead to vitreous hemorrhage and retinal detachment. Appropriately timed laser surgery can prevent many vision-threatening complications in these patients. Patients with sickle cell anemia should have baseline ophthalmologic evaluation especially with new-onset floaters or visual loss.

THYROID DISEASE

Graves disease, or thyroid-related orbitopathy (TRO), is an example of an important autoimmune disease that may have ocular manifestations. The pathophysiology of TRO is an autoantibody-mediated enlargement of the extraocular muscles, orbital fat, and lacrimal gland. A common clinical feature of thyroid eye disease is retraction of the upper and lower eyelid, with upper-lid lag on downgaze. Thyroid eye disease is also the most common cause of unilateral or bilateral protrusion of the globes, or exophthalmos, in adults. Exophthalmos (proptosis) in combination with retraction of the eyelids may produce an appearance referred to as *thyroid stare* (Figure 8.9).

Both eyelid retraction and exophthalmos may result in corneal exposure and drying, causing the patient to complain of a foreign-body sensation and tearing. These bothersome symptoms usually can be relieved by the frequent instillation of over-the-counter artificial-tear preparations and the application of lubricating eye ointment at night. The eyelid edema and conjunctival vascular congestion that sometimes accompany thyroid eye disease usually do not require therapy unless they are severe and persistent. Proptosis causing major complications such as severe exposure keratopathy or severe cosmetic compromise may be surgically treated.

Thyroid eye disease may cause other serious complications requiring an ophthalmologist's care. Diplopia due to extraocular muscle involvement is common and may require strabismus surgery. Compression of the optic nerve within the orbit can cause loss of vision, necessitating surgery to decompress the orbit or irradiation to reduce the inflammatory swelling of the muscles.

SARCOIDOSIS AND OTHER INFLAMMATORY AND AUTOIMMUNE CONDITIONS

Sarcoidosis is a chronic autoimmune disease causing inflammatory changes of various organ systems, including the eye. Ocular manifestations are characterized histologically by the presence of focal noncaseating granulomas. Sarcoidosis is most common in African American women ages 20 to 40. Laboratory findings include increased serum calcium (12% of patients), elevated angiotensin-converting enzyme (75% of patients), and abnormal chest x-ray findings including hilar lymphadenopathy (80% of patients).

Important histopathologic information also can be obtained from ocular tissues. The easiest tissue from which to obtain a biopsy specimen is the conjunctiva, but tissue from the lacrimal gland may be obtained, as it is also a frequent locus of granulomatous infiltration. Both of these biopsy procedures can be performed under local anesthesia; these areas should be considered before performing potentially more complicated mediastinal or transbronchial biopsies of lymph nodes.

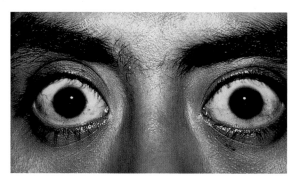

FIGURE 8.9 Thyroid stare. The staring appearance of this patient is due to forward protrusion of the eyes and retraction of the eyelids, exposing white sclera above and below the limbus.

Ocular involvement from sarcoidosis may be asymptomatic, and patients suspected of sarcoidosis should have a complete ophthalmic evaluation. Sarcoidosis may cause anterior or posterior uveitis.

Anterior uveitis is inflammation of the iris and ciliary body (Figure 8.10); posterior uveitis is inflammation of the choroid. Early initiation of topical or systemic corticosteroids is effective and may prevent complications, such as glaucoma, cataract, and adhesions of the iris to the lens, referred to as *posterior synechiae*.

Involvement of the retina is usually associated with posterior uveitis and may include perivasculitis (eg, frosted-branch angiitis or "candle wax drippings"), retinal hemorrhages, and neovascularization of the peripheral retina.

Involvement of the central nervous system is twice as common when the fundus is involved, increasing from 10% or 15% to between 20% and 30%. Ophthalmic manifestations of neurosarcoidosis include optic neuropathy, oculomotor abnormalities (including sixth nerve palsy), and, rarely, chiasmal and retrochiasmal visual field loss.

Other autoimmune or rheumatological conditions such as systemic lupus erythematosis (SLE), polyarteritis nodosa, and Wegener granulomatosis may also cause various ocular manifestations such as sclerokeratitis, uveitis, optic neuropathy, and retinal vasculitis, the latter of which may be indicated by the presence of multiple cotton-wool spots.

Juvenile rheumatoid arthritis is an important childhood autoimmune condition with ocular manifestations. About 10% of all juvenile rheumatoid arthritis patients have iritis, but the inflammation is more common with the pauciarticular form of the disease (20% to 30% of patients) and much less common in the polyarticular form. Patients who have juvenile rheumatoid arthritis, especially the pauciarticular form, require visits to the ophthalmologist every 3 months because the iritis is commonly asymptomatic. If inflammation is not recognized, extensive ocular complications may arise, including cataract, glaucoma, and calcification of the cornea.

Iritis is also a common complication of ankylosing spondylitis (10% to 15% of affected patients), Reiter syndrome, and Behçet syndrome. The latter may also cause progressive occlusive retinal vasculitis and necrosis.

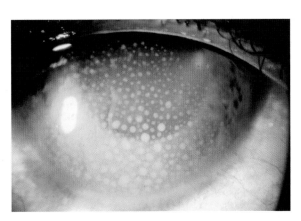

FIGURE 8.10 Anterior uveitis. Inflammatory cells collect on the inner surface of the cornea, producing opacities called keratic precipitates.

DRY EYE SYNDROME

Dry eye caused by reduced tear production may be seen in sarcoidosis because of lacrimal gland infiltration, but it also occurs in a variety of rheumatological conditions and is referred in these cases as keratitis sicca. The most common are Sjögren syndrome, SLE, and rheumatoid arthritis. Dry eye also is common in a mild form in healthy individuals over age 40. Symptoms include foreign-body sensation or burning or grittiness of the eyes, especially late in the day. Accumulation of mucus on the eyelids also occurs during sleep and is noticed by affected patients upon awakening. Many patients complain of tearing, presumably after the eye becomes dry enough to stimulate reflex tearing.

Treatment includes the application of artificial tears and occasionally lubricating ointment at night. In the vast majority of patients, the condition is annoying but rarely leads to serious ocular problems. Punctal occlusion by an ophthalmologist may be necessary. Patients with advanced rheumatoid arthritis occasionally develop severe drying of eyes and have a greater risk of corneal melting and possible perforation. In addition, they have a greater risk of corneal infection.

MALIGNANCY

Cancer originating within the eye or ocular adnexa is rare. More often, the eye is affected secondarily by cancer or by the various forms of cancer therapy. Ocular and orbital metastases are found in up to 5% of cancer patients at autopsy, most often from the breast or the lung. Usually, the tumors infiltrate the choroid, but on rare occasions the optic nerve as well as the extraocular muscles may be affected.

Systemic lymphoma affects the eye in about 3% of patients by infiltrating the conjunctiva or the orbit and causing proptosis or limitation of extraocular movement. Primary ocular or central nervous system large cell lymphoma can "masquerade" in the elderly patient as a chronic, often steroid-dependent uveitis or, more specifically, vitritis. Subretinal gray-whitish plaques at the level of the retinal pigment epithelium may accompany the vitritis and help to make the difficult diagnosis of lymphoma.

In children, leukemic infiltration of ocular tissues can occur. More than 75% of leukemia patients seen at autopsy have ocular adnexal metastases. Commonly, patients with leukemia develop intraretinal, preretinal, or subconjunctival hemorrhages as a result of thrombocytopenia or the effects of transfusion on normal clotting.

Cancer may have remote effects on the eye including autonomic dysfunction of the pupils as well as a rare but devastating paraneoplastic retinal degeneration that has a presumed autoimmune pathogenesis (eg, cancer-associated retinopathy and melanoma-associated retinopathy).

Radiation of tumors in the vicinity of the eye may lead to the development of cataract. The lens is susceptible to doses of radiation in the range of 2000 rads. Radiation damage causes a delayed retinal vasculopathy (similar to diabetic retinopathy) and optic neuropathy, typically with dosages greater than 2000 to 3000 rads and usually at least 1 year after exposure.

A variety of cancer chemotherapeutic agents have secondary ocular effects. Superficial keratitis may be caused by cytosine arabinoside, optic neuropathy may occur with vincristine injections, and retinal artery occlusion may be caused by carotid artery injection of BCNU (carmustine). Mucosal damage from graft-versus-host disease may involve the conjunctiva, leading to dryness and corneal decompensation with subsequent infection.

ACQUIRED IMMUNODEFICIENCY SYNDROME

Acquired immunodeficiency syndrome (AIDS) is a severe disorder in which depression of the immune system results in the development of multiple opportunistic infections and malignancies. Ophthalmic examination may confirm the diagnosis. Common ophthalmic manifestations are cotton-wool spots (AIDS retinopathy), cytomegalovirus retinitis, and Kaposi sarcoma affecting the eyelids. The less common complications include herpes zoster (shingles), herpes simplex keratitis, conjunctival microangiopathy, luetic and toxoplasmic uveitis and retinitis, and visual field defects or oculomotor dysfunction resulting from central nervous system involvement.

Retinal cotton-wool spots (Figure 8.11) are due to the focal occlusions of precapillary retinal arterioles that result in axoplasmic stasis of the retinal nerve fiber axons. In AIDS, the occlusions are thought to be due to microthrombi from antigen-antibody complexes and fibrin. These are frequently the sole ocular finding in patients with AIDS (more than 50%).

Intraretinal hemorrhages may also be found in HIV retinopathy, similar to diabetic retinopathy. Intraretinal hemorrhages with white centers are more atypical and may be found in other conditions such as subacute bacterial endocarditis, leukemia, and retinopathy of prematurity.

Cytomegalovirus (CMV) retinitis (Figure 8.12), an opportunistic retinal infection, is the leading cause of visual loss in patients with AIDS. The distinctive ophthalmoscopic appearance of CMV retinitis is characterized by sectoral hemorrhagic necrosis of the retina, typically along a retinal vessel. Areas of involved retina have

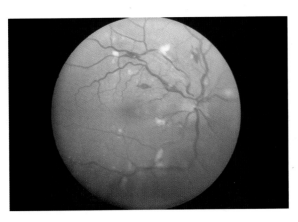

FIGURE 8.11 Cotton-wool spots in AIDS. Scattered cotton-wool spots, as well as some hemorrhages, are evident in this retina of a patient with AIDS.

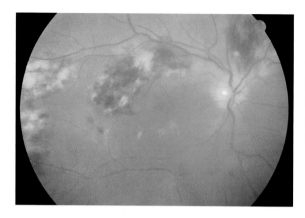

FIGURE 8.12 Cytomegalovirus retinitis in AIDS. The multicentric retinitis is characterized by discrete, fluffy, white retinal necrosis, with retinal hemorrhages and vasculitis. There is a sharp, distinct border between the diseased retina and the normal retina.

distinct borders and abruptly abut areas of normal retina. The disease progresses over weeks to months and results in total atrophy of the affected retina.

With the advent of highly active antiretroviral therapy, the incidence of opportunistic infections has decreased. Patients who can sustain a CD4 count of greater than 50 cells/mm³ are less likely to develop CMV retinitis, although higher CD4 counts are not fully protective. Most patients who develop CMV retinitis have a poorer prognosis for survival.

Both intravenous ganciclovir and foscarnet are effective treatments, but they have significant systemic toxicity including bone marrow suppression with the former and renal insufficiency with the latter. Oral valganciclovir has improved bioavailability and may be used as induction or maintenance therapy. The sustained-release ganciclovir device is a surgically implanted local alternative that continually releases ganciclovir over 8 months before needing to be replaced.

Kaposi sarcoma, characterized by multiple vascular skin malignancies, may involve the conjunctiva of either the eyelid or the globe. Unless suspected, this sarcoma may be misdiagnosed as a subconjunctival hemorrhage or a hemangioma.

In the past, therapeutic intervention was aimed at directly targeting and halting progression of the opportunistic infection. However, immune reconstitution with a "cocktail" of protease inhibitors has allowed some patients resolution of their opportunistic infection.

Any patient with a diagnosis of HIV infection should be referred to an ophthalmologist for a complete ophthalmologic examination. Detailed discussion of therapeutic intervention is beyond the scope of this book. However, when such intervention is indicated, many variables must be considered; and it is important that good communication be established among all of the patient's treating physicians and that therapy be determined based on a team approach.

SYPHILIS

Intraocular inflammation due to syphilis can be cured. Delay in diagnosis of syphilitic chorioretinitis can lead to permanent visual loss that can be avoided with early treatment.

Acute interstitial keratitis with keratouveitis occurs in patients with congenital syphilis between the ages of 5 and 25 years. It is bilateral in congenital disease and unilateral if acquired. It is believed to be an allergic response to *Treponema pallidum* in the cornea. Symptoms and signs include intense pain and photophobia and a diffusely opaque cornea with vision reduced, even to light perception. Blood vessels invade the cornea, and when they meet in the center of the cornea after several months, the inflammation subsides and the cornea partially clears. Late stages show deep ghost (nonperfused) stromal vessels and opacities. Any patient with syphilitic uveitis should have a spinal fluid examination.

Ocular involvement in secondary syphilis may feature pain, redness, or photophobia, or blurred vision and floaters. The patient may present with iritis, retinitis, choroiditis, or papillitis. There may be exudates around the disc and along the retinal arterioles in secondary syphilis and a retinal vasculitis may occur. In latent syphilis, the presenting ocular complaint is usually blurred vision. The presence of placoid chorioretinitis (ie, a circular area of chorioretinal whitening with associated subretinal fluid) usually indicates cerebrospinal fluid involvement or neurosyphilis. Diffuse neuroretinitis with papillitis and periarterial sheathing may also occur. Systemic penicillin is curative. Patients with ocular disease should receive the neurosyphilis intravenous regimen of penicillin dosing even if the cerebrospinal fluid is normal.

OTHER SYSTEMIC INFECTIONS

Other systemic infections may affect the eye. The most common are candidiasis and herpes zoster. The typical *Candida* lesion is a fluffy, white-yellow, superficial retinal infiltrate that may lead to the rapid development of overlying vitreous haze and eventual vitritis. Rarely, inflammation of the anterior chamber occurs. The presence of ocular candidiasis is a specific indication for systemic therapy with amphotericin B; intravitreal amphotericin or voriconazole may also be necessary.

Herpes zoster ophthalmicus (Figure 8.13), from varicella zoster involving the ophthalmic division of the fifth cranial nerve, may result in ocular manifestations, especially when vesicles appear on the tip of the nose from extension along the

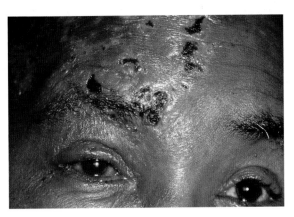

FIGURE 8.13 Herpes zoster ophthalmicus. Crusting lesions (no longer vesicles) are present in the distribution of the ophthalmic division of the fifth cranial nerve. The conjunctiva is red and the lids are swollen, indicating ocular involvement by herpes zoster. (Fluorescein has been instilled.)

nasociliary branch (Hutchinson sign). Corneal infiltration with the virus may lead to disruption of the epithelium best seen with fluorescein dye staining of the cornea. However, the epithelium usually heals spontaneously and rapidly.

Other ocular complications of herpes zoster include anterior uveitis, which can be confirmed by slit-lamp examination. The combination of anterior uveitis and keratitis, especially with loss of normal corneal sensation, is a serious vision-threatening effect. Affected patients should be referred to an ophthalmologist immediately for assistance in diagnosis and treatment. Patients can also present with anterior uveitis from herpes zoster without associated skin lesions.

Rare ocular complications of herpes zoster include diplopia secondary to oculomotor nerve involvement, optic neuritis, and retinitis referred to as acute retinal necrosis (ARN). ARN is an ocular emergency requiring emergent systemic acyclovir or intravitreal ganciclovir therapy to decrease the risk of blindness.

POINTS TO REMEMBER

- To recognize many ocular manifestations of systemic disease, the primary care physician must perform a thorough fundus examination, preferably through dilated pupils.
- Optimal blood sugar and blood pressure control may slow the development and progression of diabetic retinopathy.
- Early diagnosis of diabetic retinopathy is crucial to the ultimate success of treatment, which is effective for both nonproliferative and proliferative stages of the disease when patients are referred in a timely fashion.
- Any patient with an autoimmune disease or systemic infection who presents with a red eye, decreased vision, photophobia, or floaters should be referred to an ophthalmologist for comprehensive slit-lamp and dilated fundus examination to look for all manifestations of intraocular inflammation.

SAMPLE PROBLEMS

1. An adult patient with a 10-year history of non–insulin-dependent diabetes comes to your office for the first time, having recently moved from another state. She tells you that she has never seen an ophthalmologist nor had a dilated ophthalmoscopic examination. Her visual acuity is normal, but on dilated fundus examination, you find neovascularization of the optic disc. How do you manage this patient?

   Answer: Although this patient's visual acuity is normal, neovascularization of the optic disc is diagnostic of proliferative diabetic retinopathy, which places this patient at high risk for developing marked visual loss. She should be referred immediately to an ophthalmologist for examination and treatment. Panretinal photocoagulation laser surgery can be initiated to reverse the course of the neovascularization and reduce the risk of serious visual loss.

2. A 45-year-old man comes to your office complaining of headaches and nose-bleeds. His blood pressure is 180/120 mm Hg. On dilated fundus examination, you find numerous exudates, flame-shaped hemorrhages, cotton-wool spots, and severe attenuation of the arterioles. You do not find A/V crossing changes, and the arteriolar light reflex is normal. What information does your ophthalmoscopic examination provide about the chronicity of the patient's systemic hypertension.

    Answer: Flame-shaped hemorrhages and cotton-wool spots are ophthalmoscopic changes indicative of acute, severe hypertension. When these features occur in the absence of arteriolar sclerotic changes (ie, A/V crossing phenomenon), the hypertension is most likely of recent onset. In such cases, hypertension may be associated with renal insufficiency, encephalopathy, and impairment of cardiac function. Controlled reduction of blood pressure should be initiated immediately, with referral to an ophthalmologist once blood pressure control has been established.

3. A previously healthy 40-year-old woman presents with bilateral proptosis and lid retraction, but she denies any pain. The most likely diagnosis is

    a. Metastatic tumor to orbit
    b. Orbital cellulitis
    c. Orbital pseudotumor
    d. Thyroid eye disease
    e. Carotid artery–cavernous sinus fistula

    Answer: d. Thyroid eye disease is the most common cause of unilateral or bilateral proptosis in adults. Thyroid eye disease can be present with normal thyroid function. Orbital pseudotumor usually causes pain, whereas thyroid eye disease does not. Orbital cellulitis usually presents with swollen, tender, erythematous lids, malaise, and elevated white blood cell count. Carotid–cavernous sinus fistula causing proptosis is more common following trauma and is not associated with lid retraction, and often a bruit can be auscultated with the stethoscope over the orbit. Metastatic tumor of the orbit would not likely be bilateral with a negative past medical history.

4. A 32-year-old HIV-positive man visits your clinic with complaints of decreased vision and floaters in his left eye for the past 2 weeks. On your exam, you note retinal hemorrhages and areas of white retinal opacification. What is your diagnosis and treatment plan?

    Answer: The most likely diagnosis is CMV retinitis. Toxoplasmosis and *Candida* retinitis could also be considered, although hemorrhage is not a prominent finding in these conditions. The patient probably has a CD4 count of less than 50 cell/mm^3. He needs prompt referral to an ophthalmologist to confirm the diagnosis. Systemic treatment for CMV should be instituted.

ANNOTATED RESOURCES

Benson WE, Brown GC, Tasman WS. *Diabetes and Its Ocular Complications*. Philadelphia, PA: WB Saunders Co; 1988. A thorough discussion of the many ocular complications of diabetes.

Bhatnagar A, Ghauri AJ, Hope-Ross M, Lip PL. Diabetic retinopathy in pregnancy. *Curr Diabetes Rev*. 2009;5:151–156.

Bianciotto C, Demirci H, Shields CL, Eagle RC Jr, Shields JA. Metastatic tumors to the eyelid: report of 20 cases and review of the literature. *Arch Ophthalmol*. 2009;127:999–1005.

Bonfioli AA, Orefice F. Sarcoidosis. *Semin Ophthalmol*. 2005;20:177–182.

Boulos PR, Hardy I. Thyroid-associated orbitopathy: a clinicopathologic and therapeutic review. *Curr Opin Ophthalmol*. 2004;15:389–400.

DellaCroce JT, Vitale AT. Hypertension and the eye. *Curr Opin Ophthalmol*. 2008;19:493–498.

Kedhar SR, Jabs DA. Cytomegalovirus retinitis in the era of highly active antiretroviral therapy. *Herpes*. 2007;14:66–71.

Kotaniemi K, Savolainen A, Karma A, Aho K. Recent advances in uveitis of juvenile idiopathic arthritis. *Surv Ophthalmol*. 2003;48:489–502.

Liesegang TJ. Herpes zoster ophthalmicus natural history, risk factors, clinical presentation, and morbidity. *Ophthalmology*. 2008;115(2 Suppl):S3–12.

Mandava N, Yannuzzi LA. Hypertensive retinopathy. In: Regillo CD, Brown GC, Flynn HW Jr, eds. *Vitreoretinal Disease: The Essentials*. New York, NY: Thieme Medical Publishers; 1999:193–196.

Mohamed Q, Gillies MC, Wong TY. Management of diabetic retinopathy: a systematic review. *JAMA*. 2007;298:902–916.

Paulus YM, Gariano RF. Diabetic retinopathy: a growing concern in an aging population. *Geriatrics*. 2009;64:16–20.

Trobe JD. *The Physician's Guide to Eye Care*. 3rd ed. San Francisco, CA: American Academy of Ophthalmology; 2006. A brief but comprehensive resource covering the principal clinical ophthalmic problems that nonophthalmologist physicians are likely to encounter, organized for practical use by practitioners.

Drugs and the Eye

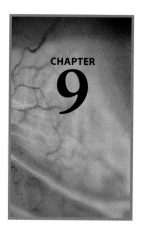

OBJECTIVES

As a primary care physician, you should be able to use pharmacologic agents to facilitate an eye examination, including staining the corneal surface with fluorescein, anesthetizing the cornea with a topical anesthetic, and dilating the pupil with 1 or more mydriatic drugs. You should be aware of the potential ocular complications of the eye drops and systemic drugs that you prescribe and be able to recognize these complications when they occur. In addition, you should be cognizant of the systemic effects of the topical ophthalmic drugs that an ophthalmologist might prescribe for your patients. To achieve these objectives, you should learn

> ➤ The technique of applying drugs to the conjunctival fornix
> ➤ The ocular effects and complications of common topical ocular drugs used for diagnosis and therapy, such as anesthetics, mydriatics, decongestants, antibiotics, and anti-inflammatory agents
> ➤ The systemic side effects of glaucoma medications: beta-adrenergic blockers, cholinergic stimulators, alpha-2 adrenoreceptor agonists, adrenergic stimulators, prostaglandin analogues, and carbonic anhydrase inhibitors
> ➤ The ocular side effects of systemically administered amiodarone, bisphosphanates, chloroquines, chlorpromazine, corticosteroids, digitalis, diphenylhydantoin, ethambutol, HMG-CoA reductase inhibitors (statins), rifabutin, sildenafil, tamoxifen, tamsulosin, thioridazine, and topiramate

RELEVANCE

You will need to use diagnostic drugs to perform a complete ocular examination, which entails skills that every primary care physician should possess. You must be familiar with the side effects and complications of diagnostic and therapeutic drugs to minimize the potential for problems and to recognize them when they do occur. (See Table 9.1 for a summary of common topical ocular drugs for diagnosis and treatment.)

TABLE 9.1 Summary of Selected Topical Ocular Drugs[a]

CLASS	COMPOUND (BRAND NAME)	COMMENT
Diagnostic		
Fluorescein dye	Sodium fluorescein	Helpful in detecting abrasions of the corneal surface. Contact lenses should be removed before instillation.
Anesthetics	Proparacaine hydrochloride 0.5% Tetracaine 0.5%	Surface-active compounds. Patients should not rub their eyes for at least 10 minutes after receiving to avoid inadvertent abrasions. Never prescribed for repeated use.
Mydriatics (dilators)	Cholinergic-blocking drugs: Tropicamide 0.5% or 1% Cyclopentolate hydrochloride 0.5%, 1%, or 2% Homatropine hydrobromide 2% or 5%	Dilation by paralyzing the iris sphincter.
	Adrenergic-stimulating drugs: Phenylephrine hydrochloride 2.5% or 10%	Dilation by stimulating the pupillary dilator muscle.
Therapeutic		
Decongestants	Naphazoline hydrochloride 0.012% Phenylephrine hydrochloride 0.12% Tetrahydrozaline hydrochloride 0.05%	Designed to temporarily whiten the conjunctiva through their vasoconstrictor effect. Chronic use can result in rebound hyperemia. Available over the counter.
Relief of allergic conjunctivitis	Azelastine (Optivar)	Antihistamine.
	Cromolyn (Crolom)	Mast-cell stabilizer.
	Epinastine (Elestat)	Antihistame/mast-cell stabitizer.
	Ketotifen (Zaditor)	Acts as a mast-cell stabilizer and decreases eosinophil chemotaxis. Available over the counter.
	Lodoxamide (Alomide)	Mast-cell stabilizer.
	Naphazoline/antazoline drops (Vasocon-A)	Provides decongestant action, antihistamine effects. Available over the counter.
	Naphazoline/pheniramine drops (Naphcon-A, Opcon-A)	Antihistamine. Available over the counter
	Nedocromil (Alocril)	Antihistamine/mast-cell stabilizer.
	Olopatadine (Patanol, Pataday)	Antihistamine/mast-cell stabilizer.
	Pemirolast (Alamast)	Mast-cell stabilizer.

TABLE 9.1 Summary of Selected Topical Ocular Drugs[a] *(continued)*

CLASS	COMPOUND (BRAND NAME)	COMMENT
Anti-inflammatory agents, nonsteroidal[b]	Diclofenac (Voltaren) Ketorolac (Acular) Flurbiprofen (Ocufen)	Used alone, these may not be potent enough to control significant ocular inflammation.
Relief of dry eye symptoms	Over-the-counter lubricant eye drops	Preservative-free formulations should be used when drops are required more than 6 times a day.
	Cyclosporine A (Restasis)	May provide relief for chronic moderate-to-severe disease.
Antibiotics	Erythromycin Sulfacetamide Aminoglycosides Fluoroquinolones	Often used to treat common bacterial conjunctivitis.
Antiviral agents	Trifluridine (Viroptic)	Topical antiviral agents should be used only under the direction of an ophthalmologist; long-term use may be toxic to the cornea.

[a] See text for additional information. Before administering any medication, always ask patient about possible allergies.
[b] Although corticosteroids are used in treating various ocular conditions, they should never be prescribed by a primary care physician; see Chapter 4 for information about the possible complications.

BASIC INFORMATION

Using the proper technique to instill eye drops ensures maximum patient cooperation and adequate delivery of medication to the eye. To instill topical ocular medications, follow these steps:

1. Wash your hands; wear disposable gloves if desired.
2. Instruct the seated patient to tilt the head back and to look up.
3. Expose the palpebral conjunctiva by gently pulling downward on the skin over the cheekbone (Figure 9.1). Avoid direct pressure on the eyeball.

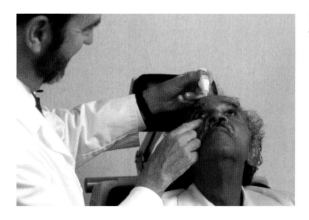

FIGURE 9.1 Instillation of topical drops.

4. Instill the correct amount of medication into the lower conjunctival fornix. Avoid applying drops directly to the cornea, which is the most sensitive part of the eye, and avoid touching the tip of the applicator to the patient's lids or eye.

5. Instruct the patient to close both eyes gently for a few seconds. Wipe any excess medication from the patient's skin with a tissue.

TOPICAL OCULAR DIAGNOSTIC DRUGS

The drugs discussed in this section are used in performing a basic eye examination and assessing certain ocular complaints commonly encountered by the primary care physician. Before administering any medication, always ask patients if they may be allergic to the agent.

FLUORESCEIN DYE

Sodium fluorescein is a water-soluble, orange-yellow dye that becomes a brilliant green when viewed under cobalt blue or fluorescent light. The dye, which does not irritate the eye, is extremely helpful in detecting abrasions of the corneal surface because fluorescein stains damaged epithelium (see Figures 1.12 and 1.13). The dye is instilled by moistening a sterile, individually packaged dry fluorescein strip with a drop of sterile water, topical anesthetic, or saline and then applying it to the inferior bulbar conjunctiva. A few blinks spread the now-visible tear film across the cornea. Although no systemic complications accompany the use of topical fluorescein, a local complication is the staining of soft contact lenses because of their porous structure. To avoid discoloration, contact lenses should be removed before the fluorescein is instilled.

ANESTHETICS

Among the topical anesthetics, the most widely used agents are proparacaine hydrochloride 0.5% and tetracaine 0.5%. The instillation of 1 drop of these surface-active compounds renders the corneal epithelium insensate within 15 seconds. Such anesthesia is useful to make surface manipulations painless, for example, to remove a superficial corneal foreign body or perform tonometry. Use of an anesthetic also facilitates the examination of a damaged cornea or saline irrigation for a chemical injury, which otherwise might be difficult because of the pain. Patients should be instructed not to rub their eyes for at least 10 minutes after receiving topical ocular anesthetics to avoid inadvertent corneal abrasions.

Topical anesthetics may produce local or systemic allergy, but this is rare. They should never be prescribed for repeated use by patients because they are toxic to the corneal epithelium; they inhibit mitosis and cellular migration and can lead to corneal ulceration and permanent corneal scarring. (See Chapter 4 for a discussion of therapeutic warnings.)

MYDRIATICS

Mydriatics are drugs that dilate the pupil; dilation may be necessary for ophthalmoscopy. The 2 classes of mydriatics are cholinergic-blocking (or parasympatholytic) drugs and adrenergic-stimulating (or sympathomimetic) drugs.

Cholinergic-Blocking Drugs

Drugs in this category dilate the pupil by paralyzing the iris sphincter. Several such drugs are in regular use: tropicamide 0.5% or 1%; cyclopentolate hydrochloride 0.5%, 1%, or 2%; and homatropine hydrobromide 2% or 5%. Atropine sulfate 0.5% or 1% and scopolamine hydrobromide 0.25% are also available for topical ocular use, but they should never be used to dilate the pupil for diagnostic purposes because their effects may last 1 to 2 weeks.

Cholinergic-blocking drugs produce not only mydriasis but also cycloplegia, or paralysis of the muscles of the ciliary body. For this reason, these drugs are often referred to as *cycloplegics*. Cycloplegia produces paralysis of accommodation (focusing), so that patients find their near vision may be blurred until the effects of the cycloplegic wear off. Nevertheless, these drugs are widely employed by physicians because they produce excellent mydriasis and the cycloplegic effect facilitates refraction.

Tropicamide is a popular mydriatic with primary care physicians and ophthalmologists alike because of its rapid onset and short duration. Maximum pupillary dilation is attained about 30 minutes after instillation, and the effect diminishes within 4 to 5 hours. Cautions regarding pupillary dilation are discussed in Chapter 1. Systemic side effects of tropicamide are decidedly rare because of its brief duration of action, but they may be serious; they include nausea, vomiting, pallor, and vasomotor collapse. Cyclopentolate produces more complete cycloplegia and is often used by ophthalmologists to perform refractions in children.

Adrenergic-Stimulating Drugs

These drugs dilate the pupil by stimulating the pupillary dilator muscle. Only one such drug is in regular use: phenylephrine hydrochloride 2.5%. One drop applied to the eye dilates the pupil in 30 to 40 minutes but has no effect on accommodation; thus, phenylephrine is a mydriatic but not a cycloplegic. Because accommodation is not affected, the patient can use near vision after instillation. However, the mydriasis produced is not as great as with tropicamide, and the pupil remains reactive to light. For these reasons, phenylephrine is seldom used alone as a mydriatic.

When maximum mydriasis is required—for example, when the far periphery of the retina must be examined—phenylephrine in combination with tropicamide is ideal because the effects are additive. This combination is often used to dilate the pupil of a brown iris as well, because mydriatics are less effective in dark-eyed individuals than in blue-eyed ones. The 2.5% solution of phenylephrine is much preferred to the 10% solution because the stronger preparation has been associated with acute hypertension and even with myocardial infarction in some patients.

In infants, the combination of cyclopentolate hydrochloride 0.2% and phenylephrine hydrochloride 1.0% (Cyclomydril) is the safest and most effective agent. Hypertension and reduced gastric emptying may occur if stronger agents are used.

TOPICAL OCULAR THERAPEUTIC DRUGS

The topically applied ocular drugs reviewed in this section are of clinical importance.

DECONGESTANTS

This group of drugs is important if only because more than a million bottles of over-the-counter (OTC) ocular decongestant are purchased each month in the United States. These weak adrenergic-stimulating drugs temporarily whiten the conjunctiva through vasoconstriction. They are advertised as effective in relieving eye redness due to minor eye irritations caused by smoke, dust, smog, wind, glare, swimming, contact lenses, or fatigue.

Naphazoline hydrochloride 0.012%, phenylephrine hydrochloride 0.12%, and tetrahydrozaline hydrochloride 0.05% are the 3 major drugs in this category. The widespread belief that the use of these compounds is part of good ocular hygiene is a misconception. Red, burning eyes may benefit as much from a cold, wet compress to the closed eyelids as they would from these compounds. Nevertheless, these agents are purchased in high volume.

The most frequent complication of ocular decongestants arises from overuse, with rebound vasodilation of conjunctival vessels. In other words, when used in excess, these preparations can increase rather than decrease redness of the eyes. In rare instances, acute angle-closure glaucoma may be precipitated in susceptible eyes by the use of sympathomimetic drugs because they can dilate the pupil. However, these drugs may be used without harm by patients with chronic open-angle glaucoma because they do not produce a rise in intraocular pressure (IOP) if the filtration angle is open.

AGENTS FOR RELIEF OF ALLERGIC CONJUNCTIVITIS

Combinations of naphazoline and antazoline or pheniramine drops are available as OTC remedies for redness and itching associated with seasonal allergic conjunctivitis. These provide decongestant action (see above) as well as antihistamine effects. Prescription medications are also available for management of these symptoms. The mast-cell stabilizers cromolyn, pemirolast (Alamast), nedocromil (Alocril), lodoxamide (Alomide), and olopatadine (Patanol, Pataday) prevent the release of inflammatory mediators and are administered chronically for prevention of allergic symptoms. Ketotifen (Zaditor) acts as a mast-cell stabilizer and an antihistamine, as well as decreasing eosinophil chemotaxis. Anti-inflammatory agents such as ketorolac (Acular) are helpful as needed for symptomatic relief.

ANTI-INFLAMMATORY AGENTS

Both corticosteroids and nonsteroidal topical preparations are useful in the management of various ocular situations. Topical ocular corticosteroids should never be prescribed by a primary care physician. The serious complications of this class of drugs are discussed in Chapter 4 and include promotion of viral, bacterial, and fungal infections as well as possible development of glaucoma and cataract. Nonsteroidal anti-inflammatory agents do not potentiate these complications. Topical ocular preparations include diclofenac, ketorolac, nepafenac, bromfenac, and flurbiprofen. These alone are generally not potent enough to control significant intraocular inflammation, however. They are also used by ophthalmologists for other specific indications, such as ocular itching, macular edema, or prevention of miosis during cataract surgery.

AGENTS FOR THE RELIEF OF DRY EYE SYMPTOMS

Millions of individuals have some level of dry eye symptoms. Palliative treatments with lubricating eye drops or ointments are available over the counter. Some patients may develop allergies to common preservatives and require preservative-free formulations. The immunomodulatory agent cyclosporine A (Restasis) is now available as a topical medication and may affect the underlying inflammatory pathology of dry eye syndrome and provide relief to patients with chronic moderate to severe disease. Cyclosporine A is relatively expensive, and an ophthalmologist should be involved in the decision to use the medication.

ANTIBIOTICS

Topical antibiotics may be used for bacterial infections of the eyelids, conjunctiva, and cornea. The choice of agent is based on the suspected infecting organism. Many commercial agents are available in ophthalmic preparations of drops or ointment.

Topical antibiotics are often used to treat common bacterial conjunctivitis. Useful antibiotics include erythromycin, sulfacetamide, aminoglycosides, and fluoroquinolones. Neomycin-containing agents, although effective as antibacterials, often cause increased redness and tearing because of topical allergic sensitivity. Antibiotics combined with corticosteroids should be used only under the direction of an ophthalmologist, because the combination may accelerate the progression of a herpes simplex or fungal infection and cause permanent damage.

ANTIVIRAL AGENTS

Topical antiviral agents such as trifluridine (Viroptic) are very effective in treating ophthalmic herpes simplex viral infections. (It should be noted that trifluridine is not effective in treating ophthalmic herpes zoster viral infections.) These drugs should be used only under the direction of an ophthalmologist, as only short-term use is appropriate to avoid toxicity to the cornea.

SYSTEMIC SIDE EFFECTS OF GLAUCOMA MEDICATIONS

The topically administered glaucoma drugs discussed in this section (Table 9.2) may have potent systemic side effects. Any drug instilled in the conjunctival fornix may be absorbed systemically by the conjunctiva, nasopharyngeal mucosa, or gastrointestinal tract (after saliva is swallowed in the nasopharynx). One class of agents, the carbonic anhydrase inhibitors, may also be given orally and may cause side effects as well. The systemic side effects of ocular glaucoma medication may be more prominent in the elderly, many of whom have multiple systemic conditions and are taking multiple other medications. The systemic side effects of glaucoma medications should be reviewed in particular with the elderly patient.

TABLE 9.2 Selected Types of Glaucoma Medications[a]

CLASS	AGENT
Beta-adrenergic blockers	Timolol (Timoptic, Timoptic-XE, Betinol)
	Levobunolol (Betagan)
	Metipranolol (Optipranolol)
	Carteolol (Ocupress)
	Betaxolol (Betoptic-S)
Cholinergic-stimulating drugs	Pilocarpine
	Pilocarpine gel
Alpha-2 adrenoreceptor agonists	Brimonidine tartrate (Alphagan P)
	Apraclonidine (Iopidine)
Adrenergic-stimulating drugs	Epinephrine hydrochloride
	Dipivefrin (Propine)
Prostaglandin analogues	Latanoprost (Xalatan)
	Bimatoprost (Lumigan)
	Travoprost (Travatan)
	Unoprostone (Rescula)
Carbonic anhydrase inhibitors	Oral acetazolamide (Diamox)
	Oral methazolamide (Neptazane)
	Oral dichlorphenamide (Daranide)
	Dorzolamide (Trusopt)
	Brinzolamide (Azopt)
Combination	Timolol + dorzolamide (Cosopt)
	Timolol + brimonidine (Combigan)

[a] Topically applied unless noted. See "Systemic Side Effects of Glaucoma Medications" in this chapter for additional information.

BETA-ADRENERGIC BLOCKERS

Topical Timolol, Levobunolol, Metipranolol, Carteolol

Nonselective beta-adrenergic antagonists reduce the formation of aqueous humor by the ciliary body and thereby reduce IOP. Timolol and its analogues levobunolol, metipranolol, and carteolol are highly effective and widely used. Because the systemic beta-adrenergic effects include bronchospasm, these drugs are contraindicated in patients with asthma or chronic obstructive pulmonary disease. Several deaths have been reported secondary to the pulmonary complications of topically administered timolol. Because of their cardiac effects, topical beta-adrenergic antagonists may precipitate or worsen cardiac failure and must be used with caution if bradycardia or systemic hypotension would adversely affect the patient.

Topical Betaxolol

A cardioselective beta-1-adrenergic antagonist, betaxolol hydrochloride, was developed to avoid the pulmonary complications of timolol. Betaxolol may be as effective as nonselective beta-adrenergic antagonists in lowering intraocular pressure. However, pulmonary effects have occasionally been noted, and caution should be used when this drug is employed in patients with excessive impairment of pulmonary function.

CHOLINERGIC-STIMULATING DRUGS

Topical Pilocarpine

Pilocarpine, a cholinergic-stimulating drug available in drop and ointment forms, lowers IOP by increasing aqueous outflow through the trabecular meshwork. Because of frequent local side effects, including diminished vision due to pupillary constriction and headaches from ciliary muscle spasm, this drop is a less popular glaucoma agent. Systemic side effects are rare, however, as systemic toxicity occurs only at 5 to 10 times the usual ocular dosage. Nevertheless, lacrimation, salivation, perspiration, nausea, vomiting, and diarrhea may occasionally occur, especially with overdosage.

ALPHA-2 ADRENORECEPTOR AGONISTS

Topical Brimonidine (Alphagan-P)

Brimonidine tartrate is a relatively selective alpha-2 agonist that lowers intraocular pressure by a presumed dual mechanism of decreased aqueous production and increased uveoscleral (non–trabecular meshwork) aqueous outflow. To date, systemic side effects of this new glaucoma medication have been few but may include oral dryness, headache, fatigue, and drowsiness, as it is lipid soluble and crosses the blood-brain barrier. Brimonidine should not be given to infants because of the risk of severe hypotension and apnea. In adults it may cause a local allergic reaction. A fixed combination of timolol and brimonidine (Combigan) is commercially available.

Topical Apraclonidine (Iopidine)

Apraclonidine, a derivative of clonidine, decreases aqueous formation and increases uveoscleral outflow. It is primarily utilized for temporary intraocular pressure control in critical situations or as prophylaxis against pressure spikes after glaucoma laser procedures, but it may also be used chronically to treat glaucoma. Its most concerning systemic side effects include promotion of orthostatic hypotension and vasovagal episodes. Locally, it has a fairly high rate of sensitivity reaction and may cause an impressive contact dermatitis of the lids and conjunctiva. Use of topical apraclonidine is associated with mild pupillary dilation, whitening of the conjunctiva, and elevation of the upper eyelid.

ADRENERGIC-STIMULATING DRUGS

Topical Epinephrine, Dipivefrin

Epinephrine hydrochloride and dipivefrin (Propine), an epinephrine prodrug, are infrequently used in the treatment of glaucoma. Epinephrine in particular may cause cardiac arrhythmia or an increase in systemic blood pressure in some patients due to its adrenergic stimulation.

PROSTAGLANDIN ANALOGUES

Topical Latanoprost (Xalatan), Bimatoprost (Lumigan), Travoprost (Travatan, Travatan Z), Unoprostone (Rescula)

This class of glaucoma medications increases aqueous outflow through the uveoscleral pathway, a supplemental route through which a small portion of aqueous normally drains. No major systemic toxic effects of these drugs have been reported thus far, but there are unique ocular effects. Patients may acquire darkening of the iris that may be more noticeable in patients with light brown, green, or hazel irides; they also may develop eyelid skin hyperpigmentation. Lengthening and thickening of the eyelashes commonly occurs, usually after several months of therapy. This cosmetic side effect is marketed in an alternate eyelash application formula of bimatoprost (Latisse), and there may also be ocular and periocular side effects with this preparation. In addition, inflammation in the eye and swelling of the macula causing decreased vision may occur, especially in those predisposed to this condition after cataract surgery or following vascular disease in the eye (eg, central retinal vein occlusion).

CARBONIC ANHYDRASE INHIBITORS

Oral Acetazolamide (Diamox), Methazolamide (Neptazane), Dichlorphenamide (Daranide)

These aqueous suppressants are the only oral drugs utilized for long-term glaucoma management. Their use, particularly on a chronic basis, is limited by a number of side effects, which include paresthesias, anorexia, gastrointestinal disturbances, headaches, altered taste and smell, sodium and potassium depletion, and a predisposition to form renal calculi, and rarely, bone marrow suppression.

Topical Dorzolamide (Trusopt), Brinzolamide (Azopt)

Topical carbonic anhydrase inhibitors lower intraocular pressure by the same mechanism as oral carbonic anhydrase inhibitors but with a much lower (but still possible) incidence of systemic side effects. Altered taste sensation is the most common systemic effect. A fixed combination of timolol and dorzolamide (Cosopt) is commercially available.

OCULAR SIDE EFFECTS OF SYSTEMIC DRUGS

The drugs covered in this section are systemically administered medications that may have profound ocular or neuro-ocular effects.

AMIODARONE

Amiodarone is a cardiac arrhythmia drug that has recently been associated with optic neuropathy. Patients present with mildly decreased vision, visual field defects, and bilateral optic disc swelling. Discontinuation of the drug may allow resolution of the optic nerve changes in some patients. Amiodarone also produces whorl-shaped, pigmented deposits in the corneal epithelium. These deposits are dosage-related and reversible if the dosage is decreased or the drug is discontinued entirely. The epithelial deposits rarely cause visual symptoms.

BISPHOSPHONATES

Bisphosphonates are used to treat osteoporosis and other conditions associated with increased bone absorption. Conjunctivitis, scleritis, and uveitis have been associated with bisphosphonate use. Symptoms include red eye, photophobia, decreased vision, and deep "boring" eye pain. In decreasing order of side-effect frequency are pamidronate, alendronate, etidronate, risedronate, and clodronate.

CHLOROQUINES

Chloroquine phosphate and hydroxychloroquine sulfate, originally used to treat malaria, are now also used to treat rheumatoid arthritis, lupus erythematosus, and other autoimmune disorders. Chloroquines can produce corneal deposits and retinopathy. The corneal deposits are usually asymptomatic but can produce glare and photophobia. The deposits regress when the drug is discontinued, but the retinopathy is much more serious. This drug-induced retinal damage is insidious, slowly progressive, and usually irreversible. The typical bull's-eye macular lesions do not become visible ophthalmoscopically until serious retinal damage has already occurred.

Chloroquine phosphate is now rarely used for the treatment of autoimmune disease due to its greater toxicity and largely has been replaced by the less toxic drug hydroxychloroquine (Plaquenil). At the standard dosages used, 200 to 400 mg daily, Plaquenil maculopathy is uncommon. All patients beginning hydroxychloroquine therapy should have a complete baseline dilated examination with visual field testing as well as color vision, fundus photography, and other testing to document fundus appearance and any other ocular conditions (eg, macular degeneration, retinal dystrophy). The exam should include counseling about the risk of retinal damage and the determination of other risks based on the patient's age, physique, drug dosage and duration of use, and any presence of renal or liver disease. Low-risk patients may be followed at a minimum 2 years from baseline. Patients at higher risk should be screened at intervals determined by their level of risk. Follow-up examinations include visual acuity, color vision, Amsler grid or formal visual field testing, ophthalmoscopic examination, and other testing as indicated. Patients on hydroxychloroquine with visual complaints should be referred to an ophthalmologist for ocular examination.

CHLORPROMAZINE

This psychoactive drug produces punctate opacities in the corneal epithelium after long-term use. Occasionally, opacities develop on the lens surface as well. These opacities rarely cause symptoms and are reversible with discontinuation of the drug.

CORTICOSTEROIDS

Corticosteroids or, more properly, adrenocorticosteroids, when given long-term in moderate dosage produce posterior subcapsular cataracts. This phenomenon has been commonly observed in people with asthma, renal transplant, or rheumatoid arthritis. Patients with rheumatoid arthritis may develop posterior subcapsular cataracts in the absence of corticosteroid therapy, but the incidence increases with corticosteroid therapy. The use of systemic or inhaled corticosteroids is associated with elevated IOP (steroid-induced glaucoma) in susceptible individuals. Oral and inhaled steroids may also precipitate or aggravate acute or chronic central serous retinopathy, a condition resulting in pooling of fluid under the macula.

DIGITALIS

Intoxication with this widely used cardiovascular drug almost always produces blurred vision or abnormally colored vision (ie, chromatopsia). Classically, normal objects appear yellow with the overdosage of digitalis; but green, red, brown, or blue vision can also occur. White halos may be perceived on dark objects, or objects may seem frosted in appearance. Usually, fatigue and weakness develop concomitantly with digitalis intoxication, but the visual disturbances often dominate the patient's complaints.

DIPHENYLHYDANTOIN

Still widely used for the control of seizures, diphenylhydantoin sodium causes dosage-related cerebellar-vestibular effects. Horizontal nystagmus in lateral gaze, vertical nystagmus in upgaze, vertigo, ataxia, and even diplopia occur with mildly elevated blood levels of the drug. More complex forms of nystagmus and even ophthalmoplegia may accompany extremely high blood levels. These effects are reversible if the drug is discontinued.

ETHAMBUTOL

Ethambutol is useful in the chemotherapy of tuberculosis. As a side effect, ethambutol produces a dosage-related optic neuropathy. At dosages of 15 mg/kg/day, optic neuropathy occurs in less than 1% of patients, but it increases to 5% of patients receiving 25 mg/kg/day and to 15% receiving 50 mg/kg/ day. The onset of visual loss may be within 1 month of starting the drug. Recovery usually occurs when the drug is stopped but may take months; occasionally, visual loss is permanent.

HMG-COA REDUCTASE INHIBITORS (STATINS)

Hydroxymethylglutaryl coenzyme reductase inhibitors (statins) include pravastatin, lovastatin, simvastatin, fluvastatin, atorvastatin, and rosuvastatin. Statins are cholesterol-lowering agents that have been shown to decrease myocardial infarction, stroke, and cardiovascular mortality in patients with coronary artery disease. Studies in dogs have shown that some statins are associated with cataract when given in excessive dosages. In humans, long-term use of these drugs has not been shown to increase the risk of cataract. However, concurrent use of erythromycin and simvastatin has been associated with increased risk of cataract. Other medications that affect statin metabolism in the liver should also be monitored.

RIFABUTIN (MYCOBUTIN)

Rifabutin is an antiviral agent used in the prophylactic therapy for disseminated *Mycobacterium avium* complex infection in patients with HIV infection and decreased CD4 lymphocyte counts. Severe uveitis has been associated with rifabutin treatment in these as well as immunocompetent patients.

SILDENAFIL (VIAGRA), TADALIFIL (CIALIS), AND VARDENAFIL (LEVITRA)

Sildenafil and its related compounds are cGMP-specific phosphodiesterase 5 inhibitors. They are used primarily for the treatment of men with erectile dysfunction. At the time of peak plasma levels, patients may experience transient, mild impairment of color discrimination, often noted as blue color tinge of vision. Mild, transient changes of retinal function as revealed by the electroretinogram (ERG) have been shown to be without significance. The ocular effects of sildenafil have been carefully studied in healthy volunteers and patients with eye disease, and no long-term effects have been identified to date. There have been a few case reports of nonarteritic ischemic optic neuropathy and central serous retinopathy, but the association with these medications has not been confirmed with postmarketing surveillance studies. Tadalafil and vardenafil are long-acting drugs and can have the same visual side effects as sildenafil.

TAMOXIFEN

Tamoxifen is an antagonist of the estrogen receptor in breast tissue. The agent is used in the treatment of early and advanced forms of breast cancer, as well as in the prevention of breast cancer. Ocular toxicity is very uncommon in the setting of long-term, low-dose tamoxifen use. Corneal changes (whorl-like opacities), inner retinal crystalline deposits, macular edema, cataract, and optic neuritis have been reported in association with high-dose tamoxifen therapy. Appropriate monitoring is indicated for patients with potential for such toxicity. Although the mechanism of the ocular toxicity is not well understood, discontinuation of the drug reverses most of these side effects. Treatment rarely leads to significant irreversible visual disturbance, and discontinuation of the drug must be carefully evaluated given the survival benefits of prolonged therapy.

TAMSULOSIN (FLOMAX)

Tamsulosin is an alpha-1a antagonist commonly prescribed for the treatment of lower urinary tract symptoms from benign prostatic hypertrophy. Intraoperative floppy iris syndrome (IFIS) is associated with the use of this medication. It is associated with a higher risk of intraoperative complications during cataract surgery, especially if it is not recognized and managed effectively. The flaccid iris, which tends to prolapse from the surgical wounds, is also associated with poor pupillary dilation and gradual pupil constriction during surgery. Other uroselective (alpha-1a) agents include alfuzosin (Uroxetral) and silodosin (Rapaflo), but there are reports of nonselective alpha-1 antagonists associated with IFIS. Cessation of the drug preoperatively does not alter the incidence of IFIS. The most important management strategy is preoperative identification of these patients and anticipation of the IFIS.

THIORIDAZINE

Thioridazine, now rarely used to treat patients with psychoses, produces a pigmentary retinopathy after high dosage, usually at least 1000 mg/day. The current recommendation is 800 mg/day as the maximum dose.

TOPIRAMATE (TOPAMAX)

Topiramate is used for the treatment of seizure disorder and has recently been shown to induce acute bilateral angle-closure glaucoma. Side effects include acute eye pain, redness, blurred vision (due to induced myopia), and halos around lights, usually within days of initiation of the medication. This association is important to recognize, as the mechanism of glaucoma is not resolved by an iridectomy, but instead with cycloplegia and topical corticosteroids as well as discontinuation of the medication. This type of angle-closure glaucoma associated with ciliary body swelling can also be seen in other sulfa-derived agents.

POINTS TO REMEMBER

- When applying eye drops, avoid dropping them onto the sensitive central cornea. Instead, release the drops into the lower conjunctival fornix.
- Never give a patient a prescription for, or a sample of, a topical anesthetic.
- Never use atropine or scopolamine to dilate the pupil for a fundus exam.

- Never use or prescribe a topical ocular corticosteroid unless you have a precise diagnosis for which the drug is specifically indicated. You must be prepared to monitor the patient for serious side effects, such as glaucoma, cataract, or infection.

SAMPLE PROBLEMS

1. A 52-year-old attorney with a history of open-angle glaucoma treated by a local ophthalmologist calls your office because she purchased some over-the-counter medication for her allergic rhinitis that has a warning about glaucoma in the package insert. The pharmacist instructed her to contact you. What do you tell her?

   a. She should never take any medication that has a warning about glaucoma.
   b. You can reassure her that she has open-angle glaucoma and there is no contraindication to this medication.
   c. She should take the medication with caution only if her allergy symptoms are severe. If she develops any eye pain or blurred vision, she should contact her ophthalmologist immediately as blindness could result in a short period of time.

   Answer: b. All systemic medications that have sympathomimetic effects can dilate the pupil. In patients with undiagnosed narrow-angle glaucoma (who have not had an iridotomy) this may precipitate an attack of acute angle-closure glaucoma. However, patients who are followed by an ophthalmologist for glaucoma would be treated prophylactically if the angles are narrow and occludable. Thus, patients who are followed by an ophthalmologist regularly with or without glaucoma are cleared to take such medications. In contrast, it is patients who are undiagnosed and unaware who may develop such complications.

2. A 65-year-old woman seeking a second opinion reports noted fatigue and decreased exercise tolerance. Her physician informed her that her heart rate was "a little slow," and she may need a pacemaker someday. A medication history reveals the use of a topical nonselective beta-blocker for the past 6 months for a diagnosis of open-angle glaucoma. Physical exam reveals a heart rate of 48 and an EKG shows normal sinus rhythm without heart block. What is your next step?

   a. Schedule appointment with a cardiologist for pacemaker evaluation.
   b. Schedule follow-up with an ophthalmologist and send letter regarding concerns with the beta-blocker.
   c. Discontinue the beta-blocker and contact the ophthalmologist regarding alternative therapy.

   Answer: c. Although topical beta-blockers are very effective and can be used safely in most patients, systemic effects can occur. This patient apparently developed symptomatic bradycardia. The beta-blocker is the likely cause and should be discontinued immediately. Many other topical glaucoma agents are available, and the treating ophthalmologist should be contacted for further follow-up and therapy. Such cardiac problems must always take precedence over chronic therapy for glaucoma.

3. A busy student comes to you during exam week because of severe headaches. As part of a complete physical, you perform a basic eye exam. During ophthalmoscopy, you cannot fully see the optic disc because the patient's pupil is very small. You find no contraindications to dilating the pupil, so you decide to do so to facilitate ophthalmoscopy. Your patient is brown-eyed, 20 years old, and has no other health complaint. Which drug or drugs would you select to dilate the pupils?

   a. Phenylephrine hydrochloride 0.12%
   b. Phenylephrine hydrochloride 2.5%
   c. Phenylephrine hydrochloride 10%
   d. Atropine sulfate 1%
   e. Tropicamide plus phenylephrine hydrochloride 2.5%

   Answer: e. The patient is experiencing severe headaches. A potential source of these headaches is increased intracranial pressure due to brain tumor, with resultant papilledema. Therefore, it is important to see the optic disc clearly to examine for these findings. Phenylephrine hydrochloride 2.5% may not be effective when used alone as a mydriatic in a brown-eyed patient. Atropine sulfate 1% is never used for simple pupillary dilation because its effects may last 1 to 2 weeks. The 0.12% solution of phenylephrine is the strength found in many over-the-counter ocular decongestants and will dilate the pupil minimally. The 10% solution is not the preferred concentration because it may be associated with serious systemic side effects in certain individuals. A combination of tropicamide with phenylephrine 2.5% usually provides excellent pupillary dilation with a relatively short duration of action and minimal systemic risk.

4. A man who has recently moved to the area is referred to you by a friend. He reports feeling especially tired lately, becoming fatigued after only moderate activity. He is also concerned about his vision; everything seems "dingy" or "yellow" to him. He's not sure when this visual symptom started. The patient has a history of heart disease for which he takes cardiac medications. Examination reveals no health problems, other than his heart condition, which appears stable. How would you treat this patient? Should you refer him to an ophthalmologist at this time?

   Answer: Symptoms of blurred vision or abnormally colored vision occur with digitalis intoxication. Fatigue and weakness are also characteristic. Usually, such symptoms occur only with overdosage and resolve with reduction of dosage or discontinuation of the drug. No other health problems exist, so it is reasonable to attribute his symptoms to digitalis intoxication. The step to take in this case is to measure the digitalis level in the blood and, if elevated, reduce the dose of digitalis. The patient should be monitored until the visual symptoms and fatigue are eliminated. Referral to an ophthalmologist is not necessary if the visual symptoms resolve.

5. A 25-year-old man makes an appointment to see you for complaints of difficulty breathing that developed after an injury. While playing basketball, he was knocked to the floor and struck his head. He went to the emergency room, where the only problem noted was a small hyphema in the right eye. He was seen by an ophthalmologist, who subsequently saw the patient for a return visit and initiated an IOP-lowering eye drop in the injured eye. The next day the patient developed shortness of breath and wheezing, and he asked to see you as he feared he may also have injured his chest when he fell. He thinks his parents told him he once had a brief episode of asthmatic bronchitis as a child, but he had previously felt this was not worth mentioning, as the condition required no chronic follow-up or therapy. What other history might be helpful for you in evaluating this patient's current symptoms? Would consultation with the ophthalmologist be necessary?

   Answer: The onset of symptoms suggestive of asthma or other obstructive airway disease after the initiation of an IOP-lowering eye drop should make the clinician highly suspicious that the patient has been placed on a topical beta-blocker. Systemic absorption of either selective or nonselective eye drops in this class may be sufficient to cause significant contraction of bronchial smooth muscle, especially in asthmatics. The ophthalmologist should be contacted to determine the exact ocular medication regimen and to inform him or her about the development of the side effects. The topical beta-blocker should be discontinued immediately, but because the IOP could subsequently rise to a dangerous level, the ophthalmologist should be consulted to determine if further ocular assessment or alternative therapy is advised.

ANNOTATED RESOURCES

Chang DF, Braga-Mele R, Mamalis N, et al, and the ASCRS Cataract Clinical Committee. ASCRS White Paper: clinical review of intraoperative floppy-iris syndrome. *J Cataract Refract Surg.* 2008;34:2153–2162.

Elson WL, Fraunfelder FT, Fills JN, et al. Adverse respiratory and cardiovascular events attributed to timolol ophthalmic solution, 1978–1985. *Am J Ophthalmol.* 1986;102:606–611. A good general overview of various ocular and systemic complications associated with Timoptic.

Fraunfelder FT, Fraunfelder FW, Chambers WA. *Clinical Ocular Toxicology.* Philadelphia, PA: WB Sauders Co; 2008. A comprehensive text about ocular side effects of prescription and over-the-counter medical agents and how to follow patients using them. An ideal reference for quick consultation.

Gorin MB, Day R, Constantino JP, et al. Long-term tamoxifen citrate use and potential ocular toxicity. *Am J Ophthalmol.* 1998;125:493–501.

Hardman JG. *Goodman and Gilman's The Pharmacologic Basis of Therapeutics.* 11th ed. New York, NY: Pergamon Press; 2001. A basic science textbook on drugs.

Marmor MF, Carr RE, Easterbrook M, et al. Recommendations on screening for chloroquine and hydroxychloroquine retinopathy: a report by the American Academy of Ophthalmology. *Ophthalmology.* 2002;109:1377–1382.

Nagra PK, Foroozan R, Savino PJ, et al. Amiodarone-induced optic neuropathy. *Br J Ophthalmol.* 2003:87;420–422.

Physicians' Desk Reference for Ophthalmic Medicines. Montvale, NJ: Medical Economics Co, updated annually. Like its the parent volume, this slim volume provides detailed data about drugs. It also includes clinical charts and tables; sections on ophthalmic lenses and specialized instrumentation; color photos, and 5 extensive indices.

Roy FH, Fraunfelder FT, eds. *Current Ocular Therapy.* 6th ed. Philadelphia, PA: WB Saunders Co; 2008. An extensive text with emphasis on drug complications.

Trobe JD. *The Physician's Guide to Eye Care.* 3rd ed. San Francisco, CA: American Academy of Ophthalmology, 2006. Chapters 6 and 7 deal with common ocular medications and ocular side effects of systemic drugs.

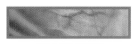

INDEX

Page numbers followed by *f* denote figures; those followed by *t* denote tables.

Naphcon-A. *See* Naphazoline/pheniramine drops
Narrow-angle glaucoma, 9, 16, 104. *See also* Angle-closure glaucoma
Nasolacrimal duct, 4*f*, 99
Near-normal vision, 12*t*
Near-total blindness, 12*t*
Near triad, 139
Near vision card, 10*f*
Near visual acuity testing, 12–13, 13*f*
Nedocromil, 184*t*, 188
Neomycin, 109, 189
Neovascular age-related macular degeneration, 61–62, 63*f*, 66
Neovascularization, 167, 168*f*
Neptazane. *See* Methazolamide
Neuro-ophthalmology
    color perception and saturation, 138–139
    definition of, 137
    examination for, 137–142
    ischemic optic neuropathy, 40, 41*f*, 153–154
    motility disorders. *See* Ocular motility disorders
    ocular motility testing, 141
    ophthalmoscopy, 141–142
    optic atrophy, 155*f*, 155–156
    optic disc elevation, 150–151
    optic nerve disease, 150
    optic neuritis, 39, 153
    papilledema. *See* Papilledema
    papillitis, 39*f*, 39–40, 152
    pseudotumor cerebri, 152
    pupillary disorders. *See* Pupillary disorders
    pupillary examination, 139–141, 140*f*–141*f*
    transient monocular blindness, 155
    visual acuity testing, 138
    visual field defects, 156–158, 157*f*–158*f*
    visual field testing, 138
    visual hallucinations, 158–159
Neuroretinitis, 179
Niemann-Pick disease, 36
Nonarteritic ischemic optic neuropathy, 154
Nonproliferative diabetic retinopathy, 166–167, 167*f*
Nonsteroidal anti-inflammatory drugs, 185*t*, 189
Nuclear cataracts, 57, 58*f*
Nuclear sclerosis, 57, 58*f*
Nystagmus, 126, 141, 150, 194

O
Oblique muscles, 4*f*, 6*t*
Occipital lobe lesion, 158*f*
Occlusion amblyopia, 119*f*, 119–120
Ocufen. *See* Flurbiprofen
Ocular irrigation, 108, 108*f*
Ocular media opacities. *See* Media opacities
Ocular motility disorders
    convergence/divergence paresis, 148–149
    cranial nerve III palsy, 145–146, 146*f*
    cranial nerve palsies
        III, 146, 147*f*
        IV, 146, 147*f*
        VI, 146–147, 147*f*
    diplopia evaluations, 145
    internuclear ophthalmoplegia, 148, 148*f*–149*f*
    myasthenia gravis, 149
    nystagmus, 126, 141, 150
Ocular motility testing
    description of, 15
    in infants and children, 123
    injuries, 104
    neuro-ophthalmology, 141
Oculomotor nerve
    functions of, 142
    incomitant strabismus caused by paresis of, 120
    innervations by, 145
    palsy of, 142, 145–146, 146*f*
Oculus dexter, 8
Oculus sinister, 8
Oculus uterque, 8
Ocupress. *See* Carteolol
Olopatadine, 184*t*, 188
Opacities, media
    acute visual loss caused by, 33
    amblyopia caused by, 19*f*, 119–120
    cataracts. *See* Cataracts
    in children, 128
    red reflex findings, 33
Opcon-A. *See* Naphazoline/pheniramine drops
Open-angle glaucoma
    aging and, 5
    definition of, 51
Ophthalmoscopy
    acute visual loss evaluations, 32
    cataract evaluations, 58*f*, 59

Vitreous syneresis, 7
Voltaren. *See* Diclofenac

W
Wood lamp, 18

X
Xalatan. *See* Latanoprost
Xanthophyll pigment, 23

Z
Zaditor. *See* Ketotifen
Zonules, 3*f*, 51*f*
Zygomatic bone, 98*f*